Foreword

Emergency medicine shares many essential elements with the core precepts of undergraduate and postgraduate medical education. Both require excellence in problem solving with the ability to rapidly assimilate and evaluate a range of medical information, participation in interdisciplinary teamwork, an understanding of systems management and an enthusiasm for meeting new, varied and unexpected challenges. Unfortunately, too often students focus their knowledge acquisition on simply passing an exam, then wonder why they have real-life difficulty in its application at the patient's bedside. Alternatively, many medical textbooks are disease-based and assume the doctor has at least reached their differential diagnosis. They rarely focus on interpreting either the initial presenting symptoms, or the basic science that underpins the physiological and anatomical manifestations of illness or injury.

This outstanding and exciting new textbook is a truly integrated work that uniquely combines real case timelines with physiological comments, clinical comments and case questions. This clever and stimulating approach with clear learning objectives will be of enormous value to a variety of learners. These include the junior medical student focusing on the physiological concepts within both the case timeline and the respective physiological comment; the more senior student and junior doctor focusing not just on these, but as well on the clinical comment to understand how to perhaps manage an undifferentiated patient; and the senior resident and junior registrar rapidly focusing on all three to now assess, treat and show others how to manage a particular case.

Here the true worth of the interdisciplinary team from the Tasmanian School of Medicine comes to the fore, with a wealth of clinical and educator experience from authors Geoff Couser, a well-respected emergency physician; Justin Walls with particular skills in medical education and as a curriculum champion; Hanni Gennat an epidemiologist and renowned physiology teacher and finally Associate Professor David Johns a respected clinical research respiratory physiologist. Their book epitomises the true essence of a spiral curriculum based on the integration of clinical data, physiological data, clinical reasoning and clinical outcomes.

This book deserves to do well, and to become a model to other writers who really want to appeal to the sense of enquiry and excitement every medical reader needs to feel when learning his or her medicine.

Associate Professor Anthony Brown MB ChB, FRCP, FRCSEd, FACEM, FCEM
Senior Staff Specialist
Department of Emergency Medicine, Royal Brisbane and Women's Hospital
Associate Professor, Division of Anaesthesiology and Critical Care
School of Medicine, University of Queensland
Editor-in-Chief, *Emergency Medicine Australasia*
Email: af.brown@uq.edu.au

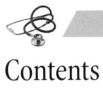

Contents

Acknowledgments

This work arose from a collaboration which evolved from developing the new five-year MBBS course at the University of Tasmania. Thanks are expressed to Professor Allan Carmichael, Dean of the Faculty of Health Science and Professor Peter Stanton, Associate Dean for Teaching and Learning, for supporting the development of this teaching resource.

The authors wish to acknowledge the contribution of Dr Jon Lane for his early support and enthusiasm for collecting material and developing cases. Thanks also to Dr Edi Albert, who, as a fellow member of the new MBBS curriculum working group at the University of Tasmania, provided many original ideas regarding integrated case delivery.

The authors are grateful to Associate Professor Tony Brown from the Royal Brisbane and Women's Hospital for reviewing the manuscript and providing valuable suggestions for its improvement.

All clinical photographs, X-rays and electrocardiograms were provided by Dr Geoffrey Couser. Consent was obtained from patients for use where identifying features are included.

Dr Geoffrey Couser's work was partly supported by a teaching grant from the Royal Hobart Hospital Education and Training Committee.

Dr Geoffrey Couser dedicates this work with much love and appreciation to his wife Kiren and son Thomas.

Dr Justin Walls dedicates this work to Tracey with many thanks for her support and work on the manuscript.

About the authors

This text has been produced by a development team rather than written by an individual. Only in this way have we been able to truly reach across the clinical–pre-clinical divide and provide a text that addresses the key problems encountered by students when attempting to make the transition from the pre-clinical to clinical environment. The development team includes a specialist emergency physician, a senior lecturer in physiology with experience in medical education, an associate professor in respiratory science and an epidemiologist with experience in instructional material design.

Dr Justin T Walls BSc (Hons), PhD, Dip MedEd

Discipline of Anatomy and Physiology,
School of Medicine, University of Tasmania
Private Bag 24, Hobart, Tasmania 7001
j.walls@utas.edu.au

Justin is currently a senior lecturer in the School of Medicine at the University of Tasmania and has gained postgraduate qualifications in medical education at the University of Dundee. He is responsible for the organisation and delivery of key medical and health science units and is playing a key role in the design and implementation of a new 5-year undergraduate medical curriculum at the University of Tasmania.

Dr Geoffrey A Couser MBBS, FACEM, GradCert ULT

Department of Emergency Medicine, Royal Hobart Hospital
Liverpool St, Hobart, Tasmania 7000
geoffrey.couser@dhhs.tas.gov.au

Geoff is a staff specialist in emergency medicine at the Royal Hobart Hospital. He is a clinical senior lecturer at the Tasmanian School of Medicine where he is responsible for undergraduate training in emergency medicine. He has played a central role in the design of a new 5-year undergraduate medical curriculum at the University of Tasmania.

Dr Hanni C Gennat BSc, PhD

**Discipline of Anatomy and Physiology,
School of Medicine, University of Tasmania
Private Bag 24, Hobart, Tasmania 7001
hannigennat@hotmail.com**

Hanni has been an active researcher in cardiovascular disease, diabetes and obesity in several capacities, including basic science, Indigenous and population health. She has a particular interest in the role of physical activity and dietary cholesterol in disease prevention and has recently been involved in a national study investigating whether biological and lifestyle factors in childhood are able to predict the development of cardiovascular and diabetes in adulthood. She has taught undergraduate physiology in medical and veterinary curricula at several Australian universities since 1995.

Associate Professor David P Johns PhD, FANZSRS

**School of Medicine, University of Tasmania Clinical School
43 Collins St, Hobart, Tasmania 7001
david.johns@utas.edu.au**

David was appointed in November 2001 as conjoint associate professor and consultant in clinical respiratory science (University of Tasmania and Royal Hobart Hospital). He is an active researcher with a particular interest in respiratory physiology, airway function and remodelling, and lung function tests. He is an active member of the Australian & New Zealand Society of Respiratory Science and the Thoracic Society of Australia and New Zealand.

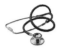

Introduction

This text is a collection of cases derived from everyday practice in the emergency department of a tertiary hospital in Hobart, Tasmania, Australia. All of the cases are real; however, specific personal details have been altered to protect patient confidentiality. Each case uses the novel approach of a timeline accompanied by clinical and physiological commentary to illustrate the links between the basic sciences and clinical practice.

The cases represent a broad range of undifferentiated emergency department presentations covering medical and surgical emergencies. Each case demonstrates the fundamental medical science of physiology, though the reader is invited to draw additional inspirations to study related anatomy, biochemistry and pharmacology. The following information is a guide for the potential users of this resource.

A guide to using the text

Each case presents the core physiological and clinical knowledge that medical students require to approach each clinical situation competently, offering an integrated approach to learning. A case *timeline*, which is summarised at the start of each case, enables students to rapidly locate relevant material. In this way each case can be viewed as a progression of basic physiological principles, with each subsequent case either addressing a different key concept, or used as a stand-alone resource for the advanced student. A clinical commentary, which runs in parallel with the timeline, provides an insight into the clinical decision-making process and a relevant context to procedures and pathologies. Similarly, the physiological commentary sections enable students in the early years of study to gain an understanding of the key physiological concepts, and enables them to understand the relevance to clinical practice. A summary of the clinical and physiological commentaries can be found at the end of each case, which provides a valuable reference and summary of the diagnosis, management and pathophysiology of the condition.

A comprehensive list of references is provided at the end of each case to act as a catalyst for further study for the student or as a resource for the teacher. Question and feedback modules are also located at the end of each case. These enable students to evaluate their knowledge and ensure their self-selected level and subsequent approach to the case material is appropriate. Further questions related to the links between cases are provided at the end of the final case study.

The layout of the text has been carefully designed to allow it to be accessed in a number of ways by the user. A series of symbols have been included in the left-hand margin to guide the students' activities while using the text.

Features of this book

- **Case timeline**: A timeline is presented at the beginning of each case and provides valuable context to the physiological content and patient management. It can be used at the start of each case to access sections relevant to the user.
- **Physiological comment**: This section indicates a key physiological concept or idea, which is central to the understanding of the case development and/or progression. Often a link will be made to how the key physiological concept informs patient management.
- **Clinical comment**: This section denotes a key clinical concept. Clinical comments are given in parallel with the timeline, providing an insight into the clinical decision-making process. The clinical comments also provide context to procedures and pathologies.
- **Case questions**: This section indicates questions you should be asking yourself with respect to the specific case. Questions of increasing complexity are presented—make sure you attempt questions that are relevant to your level of study, though you may want to tackle the next level of questions to provide additional context to the case.

Introductory, intermediate and advanced level users

Careful design and layout have enabled the presented cases to include material that is relevant to a range of end users, from undergraduate medical students to medical graduates studying for their specialist college examinations. The text has been designed to be utilised by three different levels of student, including introductory, intermediate and advanced levels. Students at each level are encouraged to utilise the text in the following ways:

- **introductory level**: presents physiological concepts in the context of the case. Users at this level should focus on the physiological commentary and use the case and timeline to provide context and meaning. This approach will lead to a sound understanding of the key physiological concepts presented in the text.

- **intermediate level**: introduces the link between clinical treatment and underlying physiology. Users at this level should approach each case from the start and work through all physiological and clinical comments in a sequential manner. This approach will enable the student to gain insight into the physiological basis of the management approach as well as the key clinical concepts presented for each case.
- **advanced level**: combines the previous levels and with a focus on patient management. Users at this level are encouraged to use the timeline as a guide to manage cases and implement decisions or tests that are of interest. Commentary on any relevant protocol-driven management approach should also be reviewed.

The three levels described equate to junior medical student (with a focus on knowledge), senior medical student (with a focus on knowing how) and registrar (with a focus on being able to show how or demonstrate). Readers are encouraged to assign themselves to a chosen level, and to then review the appropriateness of their decision by completing the question and feedback modules presented at the end of each case. If, after assigning to a particular level, you are unable to satisfactorily address more than 75% of the questions, we recommend that you modify your approach to the case material and re-attempt the self-assessment at a lower level.

A note for clinical educators

For educators involved in the growing field of medical simulation these cases provide a wealth of ideas and scenarios, which can be adapted to a number of teaching situations. The cases are all undifferentiated presentations to the emergency department. Consistent with the benefits of problem-based learning (PBL) and case-based learning (CBL) approaches, the cases present patients in real life emergency situations. For example, patients present with 'chest pain', not 'angina'; they are 'breathless' rather than presenting with 'emphysema or pneumonia'. This approach will make the students' transition from textbook theory to actual clinical practice less painful.

There are numerous applications for each case—in addition to the undergraduate knowledge and postgraduate self-study guides described above, the cases also form the foundation of a curriculum for pre-vocational doctors (postgraduate years 1, 2 and 3). Each case can be readily translated into a multi-media presentation, and the accompanying images of X-rays and ECGs are of sufficient quality to be inserted easily for teaching purposes.

Common abbreviations

Hospital departments/staff

CCU	Coronary Care Unit
GP	general practitioner
HDU	High Dependency Unit
ICU	Intensive Care Unit
RMO	resident medical officer

Equipment/procedures

ACLS	advanced cardiac life support
ACC	American College of Cardiology
AHA	American Heart Association
ATLS	advanced trauma life support
BLS	basic life support
BVM	bag valve mask
CT	computer tomography
CTPA	computer tomography pulmonary angiogram
CXR	chest X-ray
ECG	electrocardiogram
EMST	emergency management of severe trauma
ETT	endotracheal tube
FAST scan	focussed abdominal sonography for trauma
ICC	intercostal catheter (used to drain fluid from the thorax)
STEMI	ST elevation myocardial infarction

Conditions

ADHF	acutely decompensated heart failure
CAP	community-acquired pneumonia
CCF	congestive cardiac failure
COPD	chronic obstructive pulmonary disease
DKA	diabetic ketoacidosis
PE	pulmonary embolus
SIRS	systemic inflammatory response syndrome

Terminology

ABG	arterial blood gases
ACE	angiotensin-converting enzyme
ADR	adverse drug reaction
bid., b.d.	twice daily
BE	base excess
BGL	blood glucose level
BiPAP	bi-level positive airway pressure
BNP	B-type natriuretic peptide
BP	blood pressure
Ca	calcium
CK	creatine kinase
CNS	central nervous system
CO	carbon monoxide
COAGS	blood coagulation studies
COHb	carboxyhaemoglobin
CPAP	continuous positive airway pressure
CVP	central venous pressure
ECF	extracellular fluid
EPAP	expiratory positive airway pressure
FBC	full blood count; examination to look for anaemia and an inflammatory response
$FEF_{25-75\%}$	forced expired flow over the middle half of the FVC; the average expired flow over the middle half of the FVC manoeuvre
FEV_1	forced expired volume in one second; the volume expired in the first second of maximal expiration after a maximal inspiration
FEV_1/FVC	FEV_1 expressed as a fraction of the FVC
FIO_2	fractional concentration of inspired oxygen
FRC	functional residual capacity
FVC	forced vital capacity
GCS	Glasgow coma scale
Glu	glucose
GTN	glycerol trinitrate
Hb	haemoglobin
HBO	hyperbaric oxygen
HCO_3^-	bicarbonate ion
Hct	hematocrit
IPAP	inspiratory positive airway pressure
IV	intravenous

JVP	jugular venous pressure
K	potassium
Lac	lactate
LFT	liver function tests or lung function tests
LSE	left sternal edge
mane	morning
Mg	magnesium
NFP	net filtration pressure
NIV	non-invasive ventilation
nocte	night
$P(A-a)O_2$	alveolar–arterial oxygen gradient
$PaCO_2$	partial pressure of arterial carbon dioxide
PaO_2	partial pressure of arterial oxygen
Pb	barometric pressure
PCP	pulmonary capillary pressure
PEA	pulseless electrical activity; previously known as electro-mechanical dissociation (EMD)
PEARL	pupils equal, accommodating and reactive to light
PEEP	positive end-expiratory pressure
PEF	peak expiratory flow
PIO_2	partial pressure of inspired oxygen
PO_4	phosphate
PR	pulse rate
PRN	as required
PSI	pneumonia severity index
RFT	respiratory function tests
RR	respiratory rate
RV	residual volume
SaO_2	oxygen saturation of arterial blood
SpO_2	oxygen saturation of arterial blood measured by pulse oximetry
STAT	immediately, at once
TLC	total lung capacity
TPR	total peripheral resistance
U & Es	urea and electrolytes; to assess renal function and electrolyte balance
V/Q	ratio of ventilation to perfusion
WCC	white cell count
WHO	World Health Organisation
X-MATCH	cross-match

Medications

Carvedilol	β-adrenergic blocking agent
Diabex	hypoglycaemic agent (generic name: metformin)
Digoxin	cardiotonic glycoside
Dothiepin	antidepressant
Enalapril	angiotensin converting enzyme
enoxaparin	a low molecular weight heparin
Fentanyl	opioid used to induce anaesthesia
Frusemide	diuretic
Hydralazine	vasodilator
Ipratropium bromide	anticholinergic bronchodilator
Losec	proton pump inhibitor (generic name: omeprazole)
Methylprednisolone	corticosteroid
Midazolam	benzodiazepine
Penicillin	antibiotic
Perindopril	ACE inhibitor
Physostigmine	and neostigmine—cholinergic agents
Prednisolone	corticosteroid
Prothiaden	tricyclic antidepressant
Roxithromycin	macrolide antibiotic
Salbutamol	bronchodilator (β-agonist)
Suxamethonium	muscle relaxant
Thiopentone	anaesthetic induction agent
Warfarin	anticoagulant

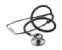

Case 1
John has crashed his car ...

This patient crashes his car and is brought to the Emergency Department in a shocked state with suspected multiple internal injuries. Resuscitation and subsequent management is directed at restoring perfusion and providing timely definitive therapy.

Timeline summary

22:30	Team prepared for arrival.
22:40	Patient arrives.
22:40–22:50	Primary survey and resuscitation, blood samples sent to pathology.
22:55	Chest X-ray (CXR) available.
23:00	Bedside ultrasound ('FAST' scan) performed and intercostal catheter (ICC) inserted.
23:10	Patient transferred to operating theatre.

Learning objectives

Physiological

- State which category of shock applies to this case.
- Understand the compensatory mechanisms brought into play by significant loss of blood.
- Describe why systolic and diastolic blood pressure are not good indicators of the severity of shock a patient is experiencing.
- Understand the physiological factors that influence the progression of shock.

Clinical

- Know how to prepare for the imminent arrival of the patient with multiple injuries.
- Understand the role of trauma systems and trauma teams to optimise care.
- Know how to prioritise assessment and management in the patient with multiple injuries.
- Understand the clinical manifestations of 'shock'.
- Understand what is meant by the term 'primary survey'.
- Appreciate the factors that contribute to road trauma in Australia.

Context

John loved his car. He loved driving fast on Friday and Saturday nights, and he loved the smells and sounds of doing 'blocks' around the local streets. Most of his friends did the same—there wasn't much else to do in his suburb on the weekend. He'd had a good week and was keen to get into town. John had a couple of drinks and was on his way to catch up with his friends. Swerving to miss a wayward animal on the highway, John lost control of his car.

His car rolled and a person in a passing car stopped and discovered him in the car, semi-conscious. An ambulance and the fire brigade were called, and the fire brigade extricated him.

Forty minutes after the accident the paramedics rang through to the Emergency Department with the following information:

'Doctor, he's 22, roll-over crash, breathing spontaneously but laboured with extensive bruising and abrasions on his right side; PR 100, BP 100/–, RR 26, GCS 11. His pupils are equal. We've inserted an IV and commenced a normal saline infusion. We'll be there in 10 minutes.'

Clinical question 1

(a) How will you prepare for the arrival of this patient?

(b) Consider your response if you were:
   (i) a sole practitioner in a remote area; or
   (ii) the team leader of a well-resourced trauma team in a tertiary hospital.

22:30 hours

The trauma team is assembled and prepares for the patient's arrival, and the team leader goes to wait in the ambulance bay to meet the patient.

22:40 hours

The patient arrives, and the paramedics report that his condition has deteriorated in the last 10 minutes. The following signs are quickly measured and recorded:

- PR: 130 bpm
- BP: 90/– mmHg
- RR: 30 breaths/min
- GCS: 10

His breathing is noisy and he does not appear to be protecting his airway. There are abrasions around the right side of his chest and abdomen and there is reduced air entry and coarse crackles on both sides of his chest. His peripheries are cool and sweaty and his pupils are equal.

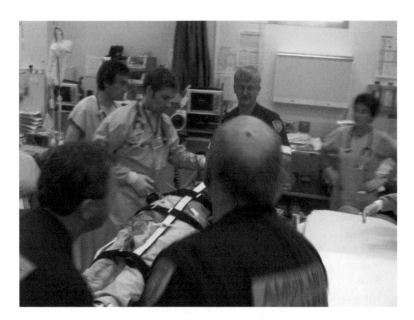

Figure 1.1 The paramedics arrive with the patient and he is moved onto the resuscitation trolley.

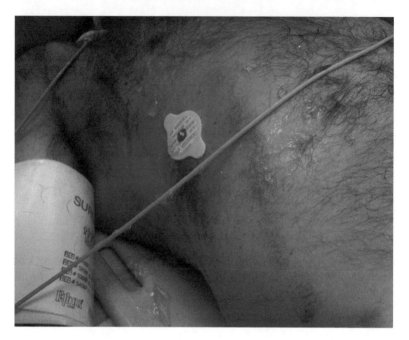

Figure 1.2 Abrasions are seen on the right side of the abdomen and thorax.

Clinical question 2

(a) What does the term 'primary survey' mean to you?

(b) What are the patterns of injury related to blunt road trauma?

(c) What are the management priorities in a situation like this?

(d) How does the emergency physician (team leader) coordinate the management of this patient?

Clinical comment

This case is taking place in a tertiary hospital with multiple staff available to attend to the patient. In rural and regional areas with few staff the sole doctor must prioritise the assessment, resuscitation and interventions. The airway is attended to first, then breathing, then circulation. This is the essence of the *primary survey*. When multiple personnel are available these priorities still apply, but they occur simultaneously under the overall coordination of the team leader. Management priorities are directed towards resuscitation, rapidly identifying the injuries and providing timely definitive therapy. Judging from the pre-arrival phone call, the patient appears to be shocked, with injuries on the right side of his chest and abdomen. Injuries such as right-sided chest injuries and right-sided intra-abdominal organ injury (such as liver and right kidney) are anticipated. This is consistent with him being the driver of a right-hand-drive motor vehicle, although any number of different injuries can occur when a vehicle rolls.

The team leader coordinates the team's activities from the end of the bed. Since they were expecting a seriously injured patient, a number of people have been notified in advance:

- surgeon;
- radiographer;
- staff in blood bank;
- staff in operating theatres;
- anaesthetist.

The team leader has briefed the resuscitation team prior to the patient's arrival. Roles have been assigned: airway doctor, procedure doctor 1 and procedure doctor 2. The doctors have read pre-prepared cards, which detail their important individual tasks. He has liaised with the nursing staff, who likewise have assigned themselves well-defined roles. The airway doctor has already decided on what personnel, equipment and drugs will be used.

Physiology comment

Shock can be defined as inadequate tissue perfusion as a result of depressed cardiac output. Shock can be usefully categorised based upon the cause of the drop in cardiac output:

- hypovolaemic (low circulating volume);
- cardiogenic (decreased cardiac performance);
- distributive (normal blood volume but vasodilation);
- obstructive (impediment to blood flow).

In this case the patient is obviously experiencing haemorrhagic shock (a subset of hypovolaemic shock). Compensation in hypovolaemic shock is often initially quite successful. Increased sympathetic outflow via the baroreceptor reflex leads to increased heart rate and contractility and increased peripheral resistance leading to shunting of blood centrally.

Remember that, even though the total peripheral resistance may increase, the resistance of the coronary and cerebral arteries may well decrease to ensure adequate perfusion to these crucial areas.

22:40–22:50 hours

The airway doctor receives a clinical handover from the paramedic, who has been applying a bag-valve-mask (BVM) device to assist with the patient's breathing. He maintains the BVM device and decides that a definitive airway is required. The patient is intubated using a rapid sequence induction. Meanwhile, the resuscitation continues.

Procedure doctor 1, a resident in the department, obtains intravenous access from the patient's left arm. She places a 16G cannula in the vein and collects blood in a 20 mL syringe. The blood tests requested are FBC, ELFT, COAGS, X-MATCH 6 units.

The doctor carefully labels the blood tubes and an orderly delivers the tubes to the pathology laboratory. A pre-prepared line of intravenous fluid is attached to the cannula; a rapid infusion of 1 litre of 0.9% normal saline is commenced.

Procedure doctor 2 has approached the patient from the patient's right-hand side. She has felt for the trachea and listened to the chest. She reports to the team leader:

'The trachea is central, there is reduced air entry and crackles on both sides, extensive abrasions on the right side … I think there's at least some lung contusion, maybe a haemothorax, but no sign of a tension pneumothorax.'

The team leader notes that:

- The airway is being definitively managed, with the patient having been successfully intubated.
- Wide-bore intravenous access has been obtained.
- Blood has been collected and sent to the pathology laboratory.
- Appropriate procedures are taking place.

However, he is concerned about the bruising down the right side of the patient.

Clinical question 3

Given the clinical presentation, what injuries do you suspect the patient has sustained?

Clinical comment

Airway

The airway doctor immediately recognises that the patient is 'not protecting his airway'. In fact, he recognises a number of troubling aspects to his airway and his breathing:

• The patient is unconscious and unable to protect his airway, placing him at risk of aspiration.
• He has noisy breathing, which suggests his airway is not patent.
• His reduced level of consciousness, in addition to suggesting a traumatic brain injury, could reflect inadequate oxygenation and ventilation.

These factors produce a dangerous situation for someone with a reduced level of consciousness:

• The patient could be hypoxic.
• The patient could be hypercarbic.

Together, these could be causing secondary injury to an already damaged brain.

Breathing

Procedure doctor 2 has recognised the possibility of bilateral chest injuries. A tension pneumothorax seems unlikely, given that the trachea is central. However, there are a number of other life-threatening conditions, which could be present and must be actively looked for. These include haemothorax, flail chest, lung contusion, traumatic pneumothorax, and mediastinal and great vessel injury. A mobile CXR is the first investigation to use to diagnose or exclude these injuries.

Circulation

Procedure doctor 1 inserted a wide-bore intravenous cannula, collected blood to be sent to the laboratory for analysis, and a rapid infusion of normal saline was commenced. This is in keeping with EMST/ATLS guidelines as an appropriate first-line response to shock.

Physiology comment

Systolic and diastolic blood pressures are poor indicators of the severity of shock a patient is suffering from. Various degrees of blood loss and the resulting peripheral vasoconstriction can lead to very similar initial mean arterial pressure readings. Due to varying degrees of peripheral vasoconstriction, patients experiencing widely differing volumes of blood loss may well exhibit similar mean arterial pressures. Therefore, the severity of shock is more reliably evaluated by other outward signs of increased sympathetic activity (pale moist skin, sweating, elevated heart rate) and level of cerebral perfusion (consciousness).

22:50 hours

It is now 10 minutes since the patient arrived at the hospital:

- The patient has been intubated.
- Fluid resuscitation is occurring.
- Chest and intra-abdominal injuries are suspected.

The patient is still sweaty and poorly perfused. The vital signs are now:

- PR: 120 bpm
- BP: 95/45 mmHg (after 1 litre of normal saline)
- RR: 15 breaths/min (ventilator settings 15 × 900 mL)
- SpO_2:   93% on FIO_2 1.0

Clinical question 4

Given the patient's clinical state, what do you think should happen now?

The team leader appraises the situation:

'The patient is still shocked after the administering of 1 litre of normal saline. I'm really worried about intra-abdominal bleeding, probably from a hepatic injury. I think we should be getting ready to move to the operating theatre as quickly as possible and while preparing to do this we should get a chest X-ray and I'll perform a FAST scan. We should also rapidly infuse another litre of normal saline and start a transfusion with O-negative blood.'

The radiographer has been patiently waiting alongside the resuscitation cubicle with the mobile X-ray machine at the ready. She moves to the side of the patient, places a film under his chest, and takes a supine CXR.

Clinical question 5

What do you understand about the role of ultrasound in acute trauma management?

Physiology comment

Some shocked patients will respond readily to treatment and seem to regain normal function quickly, whereas others will spiral down into increasing states of hypotension and ischaemia. An understanding of what physiological drivers determine whether a patient compensates and recovers or compensates and then enters into a phase of decompensation that is resistant to treatment is valuable as it underpins the clinical approach to the treatment of shock.

In haemorrhagic shock the two key variables are the extent and duration of blood loss before fluid therapy can be administered. The greater the initial blood loss the more extensive and pronounced the resulting peripheral vasoconstriction. The longer the period of vasoconstriction the greater the ensuing metabolic acidosis will be and the greater the likelihood of extensive cell damage and liberation of mediators derived from ischaemically damaged cells. Both the acidosis and liberated mediators oppose the vascular response, leading eventually to vasodilation and therefore maldistribution of much needed cardiac output. At high enough levels these factors can also interfere with cardiac function, decreasing the ability of the heart to deliver whatever blood remains to the tissues. It is vital to manage the patient so that the extent of the vascular response and the time it is experienced is minimised to ensure the best outcome.

22:55 hours

The radiographer returns to the resuscitation room and hands the CXR to the team leader, who looks at it carefully and comments:

'The endotracheal tube is in a good position, both lungs have signs of contusion and there may be haemothorax present on the left. He needs a chest tube inserted on the left.'

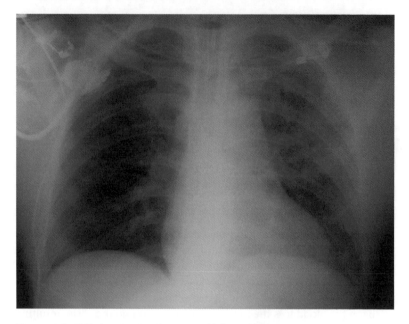

Figure 1.3 CXR showing intubation and bilateral contusion

The registrar doctor immediately prepares to insert a 32 French gauge intercostal catheter on the left.

23:00 hours

A left-sided intercostal catheter has been inserted, with 200 mL of blood drained. The patient's oxygen saturation improves, and the catheter is secured with sutures.

The surgeon arrives just as the team leader is performing a bedside ultrasound. The probe is over the right upper quadrant. The team leader points to the ultrasound monitor showing a mass of blackness around the liver region:

> 'See here? There's fluid in Morrison's pouch, I think there's a liver injury. We've only had time to perform the primary survey and resuscitate the patient, but we've got to get this patient to theatre for a laparotomy urgently.'

The surgeon quickly looks at the patient and then at the large amount of fluid represented by a mass of blackness on the ultrasound.

'I agree … I'll head up to theatre. I'll see you there as soon as possible.'

The team leader puts away the ultrasound probe.

'Right, everyone, well done so far, but now our focus is to move this patient to theatre as fast as possible and alive.'

23:10 hours

The team is ready to transfer the patient to the operating theatre. The cumbersome trolley with all its attachments and monitors and tubes is wheeled out of the door towards theatre where the surgical team is preparing for the patient's arrival.

Clinical comment

This patient is very unstable and anything other than a rapid transit to theatre is unacceptable (in the setting of a hospital with surgical facilities). A number of steps have been omitted for the moment:

- a secondary survey—this could not be performed because the patient was too unstable and the team never really got past the 'C' of the primary survey. Once the patient is stabilised further assessment can take place.
- X-rays—cervical spine and pelvic X-rays are usually part of the initial 'trauma series' of X-rays. This patient is shocked and requires life-saving surgery, so definitive therapy becomes the priority. The neck will be treated as if there is a cervical spine injury and will remain immobilised.

Bedside ultrasound (FAST—focused abdominal sonography in trauma) is being used increasingly in trauma resuscitation to look for the presence of intraperitoneal fluid. It can be a useful clinical aid in the management of these patients. However, in a shocked patient with suspected internal injuries, this should not delay rapid transfer to the operating theatre for urgent surgical intervention. Fluid resuscitation is only a temporary solution to maintain perfusion until definitive therapy can be provided. Selected stable patients with blunt trauma may be suitable for computer tomography (CT) scanning to diagnose abdominal and thoracic injury, but only in consultation with the surgical team. Unstable patients should never leave the department for a CT scan.

Clinical summary

There is more to the management of this patient than being familiar with the immediate life-threatening conditions associated with blunt trauma and the timely and effective use of primary and secondary surveys. When discussing road trauma it is essential to take a wider view and consider the major public health implications of motor vehicle crashes.

Students should consider the following aspects of this case:

- the role of emergency medical systems to optimise trauma care;
- the public health concern that injury is a major cause of death for people under the age of 44 years;
- the distressing combination of young males, alcohol and speed when considering road trauma.

Readers are directed to the references to further explore these important issues.

Epilogue

A laparotomy was performed and a lacerated spleen was repaired. The patient's vital signs improved and he was monitored in the High Dependency Unit overnight. His wounds healed well and he was discharged from hospital 8 days after his accident. He was subsequently charged by the police with the offence of driving under the influence of alcohol, and his driver's licence was suspended.

References and further reading

1 http://www.atsb.gov.au/road/index.cfm—Australian Road Safety information and statistics
2 http://www.rstf.tas.gov.au—Tasmanian Road Safety Task Force
3 http://www.swsahs.nsw.gov.au/livtrauma/—Liverpool Hospital (Sydney) Trauma page
4 http://www.trauma.org—an excellent trauma site with policies and guidance, including EMST/ATLS guidelines.
5 Kohn, M.A., Hammel, J.M., Bretz, S.W., Stangby, A. Trauma team activation criteria as predictors of patient disposition from the emergency department. Acad Emerg Med 2004 Jan; 11(1): 1–9.
6 Palanca, S., Taylor, D.M., Bailey, M., Cameron, P.A. Mechanisms of motor vehicle accidents that predict major injury. Emerg Med (Fremantle) 2003 Oct–Dec; 15(5–6): 423–8.
7 Stevenson, M.R. Steering in the right direction? Young drivers and road trauma. MJA 2005; 182(3): 102–3. http://www.mja.com.au/public/issues/182_03_070205/ste10884_fm.html

Review

Level 1: Content knowledge

1 Which of the following is not a compensatory mechanism in hypovolaemic shock?

A Baroreceptor reflexes

B Reabsorption of tissue fluids (from interstitial compartment to plasma compartment)

C Renal conservation of salt and water

D Decreased total peripheral resistance

2 Which of the following combinations would occur in hypovolaemic shock?

A Central venous pressure low, cardiac output low, systemic vascular resistance high

B Central venous pressure high, cardiac output low, systemic vascular resistance high

C Central venous pressure low or normal, cardiac output low or normal, systemic vascular resistance low

D Central venous pressure normal, cardiac output low, systemic vascular resistance high

3 Blood pressure may fall after a brief period of compensation in shock because:

A Circulating catecholamines reach such a high level that all peripheral circulation is shut down completely.

B Increased ADH secretion causes vasodilation in the later stages of shock.

C Large volumes of fluid are lost through the renal system in shock.

D The reduction in blood flow to peripheral tissue leads to the accumulation of vasodilator metabolites.

Level 2: Clinical applications

1 Which of the following scenarios would be considered to be at relatively low risk of life-threatening injury using commonly accepted trauma team activation criteria?

A A 17-year-old male has been ejected from a motor vehicle crashing at 60 kilometres per hour.

B A 33-year-old female has been in a single vehicle crash and has a blood pressure of 80/50 and a respiratory rate of 30.

C A 62-year-old male has fallen 7 metres off a roof onto the grassy ground below.

D A 26-year-old female sustains a broken arm in a low speed crash between two motor vehicles.

E A 21-year-old male is stabbed above his right clavicle but has minimal evidence of external blood loss.

2 Match the following clinical scenarios with the expected diagnosis:

A A 44-year-old female falls and injures the left side of her lower chest. She is breathless and has a tachycardia of 110 and a blood pressure of 100/60.

B A 16-year-old male is stabbed in the right side of his chest, just above his nipple.

C A 76-year-old male is the driver (right-hand drive) of a motor vehicle which collides with another vehicle. The right side of his car crumples and impinges into the cabin.

D A 27-year-old male is ejected from a motor vehicle at high speed, striking his head against the road surface. He is unconscious and has a dilated left pupil.

E A 13-year-old male is the rear passenger in a car that crashes head-on into another vehicle. He is restrained but complains of chest pain and is breathless.

   (i) Left extradural haematoma with suspected cervical spine injury

   (ii) Ruptured spleen

   (iii) Liver injury

   (iv) Pulmonary contusion

   (v) Right tension pneumothorax

3 You are the sole doctor in a rural practice. A patient with multiple injuries is brought in by the ambulance. The patient is unconscious, has signs of chest, abdominal and orthopaedic injuries, and is clinically shocked. Using the principles of the primary survey, choose the most appropriate sequence of responses:

A Decompress the tension pneumothorax, obtain intravenous access, control external bleeding, support the airway, commence intravenous fluids, splint the fractures.

B Obtain intravenous access, commence intravenous fluids, control external bleeding, splint the fractures, support the airway and decompress the tension pneumothorax.

C Splint the fractures, control external bleeding, obtain intravenous access, commence intravenous fluids, support the airway and decompress the tension pneumothorax.

D Support the airway, decompress the tension pneumothorax, obtain intravenous access, commence intravenous fluids, control external bleeding, splint the fractures.

E Support the airway, decompress the tension pneumothorax, control external bleeding, splint the fractures, obtain intravenous access, commence intravenous fluids.

Level 3: Topics for further discussion

1 Discuss how trauma is managed in your region and how teamwork can be enhanced and practised.
2 Which intravenous fluids should be used in trauma management?

Case 2
Don's wife finally convinced him to seek treatment

This 76-year-old male has been unwell for the last few months, but in the early hours of this morning he becomes too breathless to sleep. His wife insists he seek medical help, and he arrives in the Emergency Department shortly after 3 a.m. A careful but timely history and examination identifies the problem and the reason it became particularly bad tonight …

Timeline summary

01:40	Wakes from sleep breathless.
03:05	Arrives at Emergency Department; triaged category 3.
03:15	Led into a cubicle; nursing staff commence assessment.
03:30	Seen by resident medical officer.
03:30	12-lead electrocardiogram (ECG).
03:50	Intravenous access, bloods sent to pathology.
04:15	Chest X-ray (CXR) taken.
04:25	Patient and results reviewed; therapy commenced.
04:45	Referred for medical admission.

Learning objectives

Physiological

- Describe the physiological basis of breathlessness.
- Understand how rheumatic fever as a child may lead to congestive heart failure.
- Explain to what degree the heart is able to compensate for valvular abnormalities.
- Understand how congestive cardiac failure (CCF) can lead to inappropriate reabsorption of salt and water by the kidneys.
- List the factors controlling β-type natriuretic protein (BNP) release.
- Describe the physiological basis of atrial fibrillation.

Clinical

- Describe the possible causes for breathlessness in this context.
- Be able to recognise the symptoms and signs of heart failure.
- Understand the appropriate and timely use of investigations to diagnose CCF.
- Understand the acute and longer-term management of CCF and the evidence behind it.

Context

Don has been fairly healthy all of his life. He had rheumatic fever as a child, but other than that he'd been well for years. He had mildly elevated blood pressure for which he took a tablet daily. He had worked as an engineer for the local council until his retirement 11 years ago. He played bowls regularly and liked nothing better than to have lunch every day with Jan, his wife of over 50 years.

Over the last few weeks he'd been noticing that he had been getting breathless when walking up the gentle hill near his house. He thought this was due to 'old age' and that it would settle down with time. However, it had been getting steadily worse and now he was even getting puffed walking around the house. A couple of times he'd actually been woken up at night gasping for breath.

Tonight was 'one of those nights'. He'd gone to bed feeling well enough but now, just after 1:30 a.m., he felt he couldn't get his breath. His wife was woken by his noisy breathing. He assured her that he would settle down, but she realised that he needed help. Despite feeling better after sitting up in bed for a few minutes, he reluctantly agreed and allowed her to drive him to hospital. They arrived at the Emergency Department just after 3:00 a.m. Don was feeling much better by this time and when seen by the triage nurse he was given a triage 'category 3'. He was led into a cubicle where he changed into a hospital gown and waited for the nurse and doctor to see him.

03:25 hours

The department has been fairly busy for a Tuesday night and Helen, the intern rostered on overnight, has been working hard since her shift began at 10:30 p.m. Things are settling down now, and Helen has finally been able to sit down for a cup of coffee and a bowl of fruit. Feeling refreshed, she returns to the Emergency Department floor and checks to see who is the next patient to be seen.

Helen walks into the cubicle to find the nurse completing her observations.

'Here you are', she says, handing the sheet to the intern. 'Let me know if there's anything else you'd like.'

The observations are as follows:

- Elderly male c/o breathlessness. Now settled.
- PR: 86 bpm, irregular
- BP: 160/110 mmHg
- RR: 20 breaths/min
- temperature: 36.7°C
- SpO$_2$: 95% room air

Don is quite comfortable sitting on the trolley. Helen introduces herself to him and begins her assessment.

Physiology comment

Dyspnoea (breathlessness)

The American Thoracic Society defines dyspnoea (shortness of breath; breathlessness) as 'a term used to characterise a subjective experience of breathing discomfort that is comprised of qualitatively distinct sensations that vary in intensity'. Others have defined it as an undue awareness of breathing or awareness of breathing difficulty. The subjective nature of dyspnoea makes it difficult to quantify.

Dyspnoea can be caused by a range of factors, including:

- reduced oxygenation;
- acidosis;
- stimulation of a range of mechanoreceptors in the lung;
- inadequate delivery to, or utilisation of, oxygen by peripheral tissues;
- inability to respond to ventilatory demands, for example due to increased resistance to breathing, inspiratory muscle fatigue;
- psychogenic issues.

Clinical question 1

(a) Describe your approach to a patient such as Don.
(b) List the differential diagnoses you are considering at this early stage.
(c) What questions will you ask him?

Helen proceeds to take a detailed history from Don. He tells her about his breathlessness over the preceding few weeks, and how he sometimes felt as if he couldn't breathe when he was lying in bed at night and how he would feel better when he sat up. In fact, he would feel better if he slept propped up on a couple of pillows. This prompts Helen to ask some more specific questions.

Clinical question 2

(a) What are the medical terms for Don's symptoms?
(b) What condition are they suggestive of?
(c) Describe how you will proceed now.

Helen thinks that this points towards heart failure as a possible cause of Don's symptoms. She glances at his ankles, and notes that they looked swollen. She takes his pulse, and notes that it felt irregular. She looks at Don and continues to take her history.

Dr Helen: 'Have you ever had any chest pain?'

Don: 'No, never.'

Dr Helen: 'Have you ever had any problems with your heart?'

Don: 'I had rheumatic fever when I was a child and I was told it could affect my heart later, but I've never noticed anything. A doctor once said I had a murmur ...'

Dr Helen: 'Do you take any medication?'

Don: 'I'm on Diltiazem for my blood pressure. I've been on it for years.'

Dr Helen: 'Your legs seem quite swollen—has this been a problem for long?'

Don: 'Come to think of it, I've only noticed them in the last few weeks ... my shoes have become a bit tight ...'

Clinical question 3

(a) Do these answers help you make a diagnosis?
(b) What do they reveal?
(c) Are there any significant findings in this history that lead you towards a particular diagnosis?

Clinical comment

Don has fairly typical symptoms of CCF, as evidenced by his paroxysmal nocturnal dyspnoea (waking up breathless from sleep), orthopnoea (inability to breathe except in an upright position) and evidence of peripheral oedema. These form part of various diagnostic criteria in existence, such as the Framingham criteria and the WHO criteria for the diagnosis of heart failure. Of particular significance are the findings of a history of rheumatic heart disease (which predisposes to the development of valvular heart disease), the presence of an irregular pulse (suggesting atrial fibrillation) and his use of calcium channel blocker medication (which has a negative inotropic effect and may exacerbate heart failure). The role of the medical practitioner in this instance is to make and confirm the diagnosis, consider precipitants and commence appropriate therapy.

Physiology comment

Aetiology of congestive cardiac failure

It is believed to be the immunological component of rheumatic disease that causes scarring of the endothelial layer of the heart valves, which can later become symptomatic. In the disease, the mitral and tricuspid valves are often affected, along with the aortic valve. If a history of rheumatic disease is elicited, it is important to consider that often multiple valves are affected and therefore cardiac symptoms can be more complex.

Helen thinks to herself that the diagnosis of CCF is likely, but she needs more information. She performs a physical examination. She requests that a 12-lead ECG and a CXR be performed, and she proceeds to insert an intravenous cannula and obtain blood to be sent to pathology.

Clinical question 4

(a) What blood tests would you request at this stage?
(b) Discuss the role of BNP in the diagnosis of heart failure.
(c) What physical findings would you expect to find?
(d) Would you commence any treatment at this time?
(e) List the possible precipitants of heart failure.

Helen records her physical examination findings as follows (see Fig. 2.1).

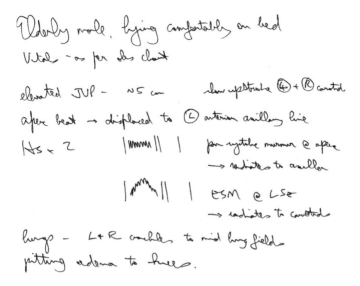

Figure 2.1 Doctor's handwritten notes

03:30 hours

The ECG is performed by the nurse and shown to the intern (see Fig. 2.2).

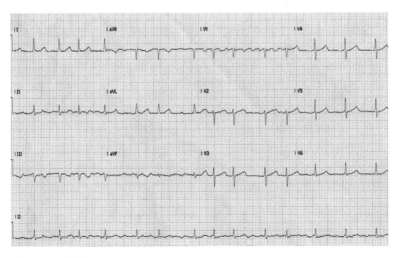

Figure 2.2 ECG

The CXR is performed (see Fig. 2.3).

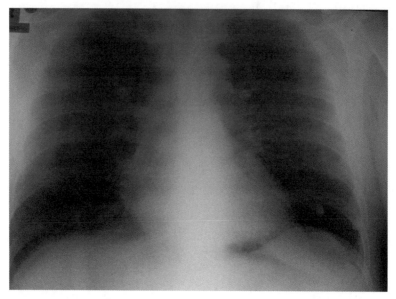

Figure 2.3 Chest X-ray

Clinical question 5

(a) Describe the ECG and the CXR as if you are presenting your findings to a colleague.

(b) Summarise the findings into a diagnosis and write a problem list. Discuss what may have precipitated the condition.

(c) Does Don require admission to hospital?

(d) If so, describe how you will refer him to the inpatient team. Include your diagnosis and initial management plan.

04:25 hours

Helen returns to the cubicle and sits down with Don and his wife.

'The results have come back and there's a good reason you've been feeling so breathless recently. You do have two murmurs, and they're contributing to your heart condition. Also, your heart is in an irregular rhythm called "atrial fibrillation". This is all causing your heart to not pump as effectively as it should, and fluid is accumulating in your lungs and the rest of your body. Your condition is called "congestive cardiac failure", and we need to admit you to hospital.'

Helen proceeds to discuss the nature of Don's condition with him and his wife, and to initiate therapy to treat his condition (see Table 2.1).

Table 2.1 Medication administered to patient

Treatment	Route	Rationale
40 mg frusemide	IV	To reduce the amount of fluid overload
500 µg digoxin—first of his loading dose	Oral	To control rate of atrial fibrillation
80 mg enoxaparin	Subcutaneous	To provide therapeutic anti-coagulation (as prophylaxis for thromboembolism secondary to his atrial fibrillation) as well as treatment for a possible ischaemic cause
150 mg aspirin	Oral	Presumptive treatment for a possible ischaemic cause for his condition
Cessation of calcium channel blocker		Removal of a negative inotropic agent which may worsen his cardiac failure
Commenced ACE inhibitor: 10 mg enalapril daily		ACE inhibitors have been shown to improve morbidity and mortality in patients with CCF
Patient weighed and placed onto fluid balance observations		To track efficacy of diuretic therapy
Request form for transthoracic echocardiogram sent to cardiology department		To assess heart structure and function

04:45 hours

Don is referred to the medical registrar for admission.

Physiology comment

Atrial fibrillation

Atrial fibrillation is an irregular rhythm generated by disorganised atrial depolarisation, with random conduction of some impulses through the atrio-ventricular (AV) junction to the ventricles. Chronic CCF is associated with atrial fibrillation due to enhanced automaticity and multiple re-entry circuits created by atrial deformation. The increased resistance at the AV node normally blocks most atrial impulses, but the ventricular rate is often in excess of 200 bpm. The faster the ventricular rate, the greater the decrease in cardiac output owing to reduced stroke volume and cardiac output. An irregular rhythm with p waves replaced with a characteristic wavy baseline (f-waves) can be observed on the ECG. The QRS complex will be normal unless additional conduction abnormalities occur downstream of the AV node.

Cardiac compensation in aortic stenosis

In aortic stenosis, a pressure gradient develops across the damaged valve as the left ventricle is forced to generate an increased pressure to overcome the stenosed opening. The patient often remains asymptomatic during the early stages of the disease, as the left ventricle is able to compensate adequately (via the mechanism of increased preload). However, as the left ventricular wall begins to hypertrophy in response to the increased pressure the reduced wall compliance decreases filling volume, leading to a drop in cardiac output. In order to maintain blood pressure, total peripheral resistance (TPR) increases. As diastolic pressure is determined by the ease of blood run-off to the venous side of the circulation, this increase in TPR often leads to an increase in diastolic pressure. Over time, usually several symptoms gradually appear:

- angina;
- syncope;
- heart failure.

Angina occurs when the coronary blood flow is unable to meet the requirements of the hypertrophied myocardium, especially during exercise. Syncope may result from an inappropriate haemodynamic reflex in which the TPR falls, thereby causing decreased cerebral perfusion. Arrhythmias and/or heart block secondary to the hypertrophied myocardium may also lead to reduced blood pressure and syncope. Dyspnoea can result from pulmonary capillary congestion (secondary to left ventricular

(LV) failure), which reduces haemoglobin oxygenation and diminishes lung compliance.

Orthopnoea refers to dyspnoea that occurs while lying and results from pooling of blood in the central vasculature due to gravity, which leads to an increase in cardiac volume. This increased LV preload leads to an increased gradient across the aortic valve, and therefore backup of blood in the pulmonary capillaries. Orthopnoea is relieved by propping the upper body up in order to reduce the venous return. Paroxysmal nocturnal dyspnoea is the occurrence of sudden dyspnoea that wakes the patient from sleep. It may occur when the patient inadvertently slips off the pillows used to elevate the upper body.

Clinical comment

Don has been diagnosed with congestive cardiac failure. He is classified as Class 3 heart failure using the ACC/AHA classification system, evidenced by dyspnoea, fatigue and reduced exercise tolerance. His immediate problem list looks like this:

biventricular CCF, precipitated by:
- valvular heart disease (likely aortic stenosis and mitral regurgitation);
- atrial fibrillation;
- possible underlying ischaemic heart disease;
and exacerbated by use of a calcium channel blocker.

Don has clinical features of left heart failure (orthopnoea and paroxysmal nocturnal dyspnoea) and right heart failure (elevated jugular venous pressure and peripheral oedema). The distinction is usually artificial, and most patients seem to have some element of both. In this circumstance he was not in acute respiratory distress, so it was reasonable to commence therapy once more information became available.

His ECG showed that he was in atrial fibrillation. Although there were no specific features of ischaemia on this particular ECG, cardiac ischaemia is an important cause to consider for patients in this age group. His CXR revealed no overt pulmonary oedema, but he had a mild cardiomegaly consistent with the clinical diagnosis of CCF.

The use of the BNP as a diagnostic aid is growing around the world. It may be of benefit in distinguishing cardiac causes from respiratory causes of breathlessness. While Don's diagnosis may seem quite straightforward, in some circumstances it is difficult to distinguish between different causes of breathlessness. In fact, many patients have concurrent illnesses, and it is not uncommon for patients with emphysema to have an element of right heart failure as well.

Congestive cardiac failure is a growing problem in Australia, and the National Institute of Clinical Studies has focused on four key areas:

- recognition of heart failure symptoms;
- diagnosis of heart failure;
- prescription of appropriate drugs, particularly angiotensin-converting enzyme (ACE) inhibitors and β-blockers;
- adherence to treatment, particularly medication.

In this case, emphasis is on the first two points. Don should notice a significant improvement in his symptoms once appropriate therapy has been commenced. He will require further investigation of his heart function and of the precipitants of his heart failure. Medical therapy may be sufficient, but surgical therapy of his valvular disease may be required. He may require long-term anticoagulation for his atrial fibrillation. These issues will need to be discussed with his treating cardiologist.

Physiology comment

Congestive cardiac failure and renal function

In the later stages of CCF the renal system often inappropriately reabsorbs both salt and water. This leads to an expansion of the extracellular fluid volume, further exacerbating the central and peripheral oedema already present. The renal system is stimulated to reabsorbed salt and water due to the reduction in blood pressure brought about by the cardiac failure. The lowered blood pressure is sensed by both intrarenal (afferent arteriolar and macula densa) pressure/flow and extrarenal (baroreceptors) receptors that bring about activation of the renin/angiotensin/aldosterone system.

The renal system has no way of directly responding to extracellular fluid (ECF) volume changes, and instead relies upon an indirect measure of blood pressure to alter salt and water balance. Under normal conditions ECF volume and total body sodium decrease and increase in step with blood pressure. In CCF, however, the link between increasing ECF volume (preload) and increasing blood pressure is lost due to the failing heart. Therefore even though the ECF volume is progressively increasing the blood pressure remains low (and may even fall if the myocardium is overstretched or damaged) and the kidney responds by increasing the ECF volume even further.

Factors controlling B-type natriuretic factor release

Cells in the cardiac atria secrete a peptide hormone called B-type natriuretic protein (BNP) when the atria are overstretched (as seen during ECF volume expansion) in CCF. B-type natriuretic factor acts to inhibit sodium reabsorption directly or indirectly by the nephron, therefore offsetting to some degree the almost total reabsorption of sodium that occurs in CCF.

Epilogue

Don spent 5 days in hospital. He lost 6.5 kg in weight, indicating that he was significantly overloaded with fluid upon admission. His echocardiogram showed significant disease of his aortic and mitral valves, and a subsequent angiogram confirmed this. The same angiogram revealed no significant coronary artery disease. He was still in atrial fibrillation upon discharge, and he had been commenced on oral anticoagulation. His discharge medications were:

- warfarin: 3 mg nocte
- digoxin: 125 μg mane
- enalapril: 20 mg mane
- carvedilol: 3.125 mg b.d.
- frusemide: 40 mg mane

He was referred to a cardiothoracic surgeon for valve replacement surgery. A nurse practitioner specialising in heart failure will visit him regularly to ensure optimal use of his medication and to identify any early signs of deterioration.

References and further reading

1   National Heart Foundation of Australia and Cardiac Society of Australia and New Zealand Chronic Heart Failure Clinical Practice Guidelines Writing Panel. Guidelines for management of patients with chronic heart failure in Australia. MJA 2001; 174: 459–66. www.mja.com.au
2   National Institute of Clinical Studies. The diagnosis and recognition of congestive cardiac failure. Prepared by the Centre for Evidence Based Practice at the University of Queensland. 2002. NICS, Melbourne. http://www.nicsl.com.au
3   Ewald, B. B-type natriuretic peptide: a new diagnostic tool for congestive heart failure. Aust Prescr 2003; 26: 64–5.
4   Talley, N.J. and O'Connor, S. Examination medicine. 5th edn, 2006. Sydney, Churchill & Livingstone.

5 Hunt, S.A., Baker, D.W., Chin, M.H., Cinquegrani, M.P., Feldman, A.M., Francis, G.S., Ganiats, T.G., Goldstein, S., Gregoratos, G., Jessup, M.L., Noble, R.J., Packer, M., Silver, M.A. and Stevenson, L.W. ACC/AHA guidelines for the evaluation and management of chronic heart failure in the adult: A report of the American College of Cardiology/American Heart Association Task Force on Practice Guidelines (Committee to Revise the 1995 Guidelines for the Evaluation and Management of Heart Failure). 2001. American College of Cardiology website: http://www.acc.org/clinical/guidelines/failure/hf_index.htm

6 Mueller, C., Scholer, A., Laule-Kilian, K. et al. Use of B-type natriuretic peptide in the evaluation and management of acute dyspnea. N Engl J Med 2004 Feb 12; 350(7): 647–54.

Review

Level 1: Content knowledge

1 The inappropriate retention of salt and water by the kidneys often seen in cases of chronic cardiac failure is caused by:
   A Increased circulating volume stimulating the baroreceptor response
   B Increased circulating volume not resulting in an increase in cardiac output and blood pressure
   C A hypovolaemic state stimulating the baroreceptor response
   D A lack of the baroreceptor response

2 Which of the following is not a cause of dyspnoea?
   A Acidosis
   B Stimulation of mechanoreceptors in the lung
   C Inadequate delivery to, or utilisation of, oxygen by peripheral tissues
   D Increased haematocrit

3 In aortic stenosis:
   A A pressure gradient develops across the stenosed valve.
   B Pressure increases after the stenosed valve.
   C The ventricle will progressively become more compliant.
   D Total peripheral resistance will decrease.

Level 2: Clinical applications

1 Which of the following therapies have proven benefit in the management of congestive heart failure?
   A Digoxin
   B Angiotensin converting enzyme (ACE) inhibitors
   C Verapamil (a calcium channel blocker)
   D Amiodarone
   E All of the above have a role in the management of congestive heart failure.

2 Which of the following symptoms are not suggestive of congestive cardiac failure as a cause of breathlessness?
   A Orthopnoea
   B Fatigue
   C Cough
   D Paroxysmal nocturnal dyspnoea
   E Haemoptysis

3 Which of the following diagnostic tests is the least helpful in diagnosing heart failure?

A Echocardiography

B Electrocardiography

C Chest X-ray

D Full blood count

E Spirometry

4 Match the following precipitants for heart failure with their clinical presentation:

A Pneumonia

B Myocardial ischaemia

C Atrial fibrillation

D Anaemia

E Severe aortic stenosis

F Obstructive sleep apnoea

    (i) Palpitations and light-headedness

   (ii) Lethargy and dark stools

  (iii) Central chest pain radiating to jaw

  (iv) Pleuritic chest pain and cough

   (v) Overweight and falling asleep at work

  (vi) Syncopal episodes with exertion and ejection systolic murmur

Level 3: Topics for further discussion

1 Discuss the role of the family doctor in optimising care of the patient with cardiac failure.

2 Discuss the evidence relating to optimal management of patients with heart failure.

Case 3
What is wrong with Mrs Jennings?

This 72-year-old patient presents with diagnostic and management challenges. After the diagnosis is made the clinical team is faced with a life-threatening situation that must be dealt with immediately.

Timeline summary

09:00	Arrives at Emergency Department by ambulance.
09:25	Assessment by medical staff.
09:50	Investigations ordered, 12-lead electrocardiogram (ECG) obtained, and intravenous rehydration commenced.
11:10	Initial investigations available and reviewed.
11:25	Initial rehydration complete; referred for medical admission and supportive care continues.
16:45	Patient suddenly deteriorates.
16:55	Arterial blood gases (ABG), mobile chest X-ray (CXR) and second ECG obtained.
17:00	Results explained to patient; thrombolysis administered.
17:15	Marked clinical improvement; computer tomography pulmonary angiogram (CTPA) arranged.
18:15	Patient admitted to Coronary Care Unit (CCU) for observation and further investigations to determine cause.

Learning objectives

Physiological

- Describe the role of the baroreceptor reflex in maintaining blood pressure.

- List the possible causes of orthostatic changes in blood pressure.
- Understand how pulmonary embolism (PE) can lead to obstructive shock.
- Explain how PE can lead to a mismatch between ventilation and perfusion.

Clinical

- Understand the principles of timely assessment and management of the undifferentiated patient.
- Understand the indications and limitations of pathological and radiological investigations in patients with undifferentiated illness.
- Know how to respond when confronted with a medical emergency.
- Appreciate the different presentations of patients with thromboembolic disease.

Context

Mrs Jennings, a 72-year-old female, presents to the Emergency Department complaining of three weeks of intermittent dizziness and a 'viral illness'. She had been brought to Emergency Department by ambulance because she felt particularly unwell this morning. She had been triaged 'category 3'.

09:25 hours

You are working as the resident in the Emergency Department. Your initial impression of Mrs Jennings is that she is sitting comfortably in bed and looks reasonably well. The following vital signs have been recorded by nursing staff prior to your assessment:

- PR: 115 bpm
- temperature: 37.7°C
- BP: 130/80 mmHg lying; 90/60 mmHg sitting
- SpO_2: 97% on room air
- appears 'dry'.

You introduce yourself and note that she appears a bit anxious: she cares for her frail husband and she is concerned for his welfare while she is in hospital. You proceed to take a more detailed history.

Mrs Jennings began feeling 'generally unwell' 3 weeks ago. She felt tired and rundown, and would often feel dizzy, especially on standing. She had not been taking much in the way of oral fluids or solids, and it had progressed to the point where she felt she could not get up out of bed. She denied any breathlessness or chest pain. She had seen her family doctor twice in the last 3 weeks; on the second occasion her antihypertensive medication had been ceased because of the postural blood pressure changes.

Clinical question 1

(a) What are you thinking?
(b) Is there anything to suggest that she has anything more than a 'viral illness'?
(c) What else would you ask her at this stage?

Physiology comment

As a person moves from a lying to an upright position the cardiac output tends to fall by approximately 20%. This fall in cardiac output would be greater except for the influence of several autonomically mediated reflexes. The decreased venous return leads to a fall in the right atrial volume, which ultimately leads to a drop in arterial pressure. Baroreceptors quickly sense this drop in pressure and elicit an increased sympathetic output that increases heart rate, contractility and total peripheral resistance (TPR). One or a combination of the following causes the poor orthostatic response seen in the above patient:

- reduced ability of autonomic nervous system to increase heart rate and stroke volume and therefore cardiac output;
- reduced ability of the autonomic nervous system to increase TPR;
- reduced total blood volume;
- misdistribution of blood volume.

Mrs Jennings has a past history of diet controlled type 2 diabetes and hypertension. She is currently taking no medication (her perindopril had been ceased in the last 3 weeks), and she is not allergic to anything. In fact, she is very fit and active and independent in all activities.

You proceed to conduct a physical examination. As mentioned above, she looks well but mildly dehydrated, and her vital signs have been noted. The examination reveals no additional clinical signs.

Clinical question 2

(a) What is your differential diagnosis list now that you have examined her?

(b) How will you proceed from here?

Clinical comment

There are some so-called 'red flags' present: she has an unexplained tachycardia and a significant postural blood pressure drop, and the symptoms have been present for 3 weeks. This woman is usually well and active, and it is most unusual for her to be lacking in energy. It could be important to ask questions relating to cardiovascular, respiratory and infectious symptoms.

You cannot find any specific findings at this stage, but you are concerned that her condition has been present for 3 weeks and that your patient is unable to mobilise and care for herself or her husband. Something must be going on, but the answer is not yet clear. The idea of 'assessment and management occur in parallel' is at the forefront of your mind as well. You feel that further investigation is required.

Clinical question 3

(a) What investigations may help you make a diagnosis? Justify your choices.

(b) What management can you implement at this stage?

09:50 hours

You request the following investigations:

- full blood examination: to look for anaemia and an inflammatory response;
- urea and electrolytes/liver function tests/Ca, Mg, PO_4: the patient appears clinically dehydrated, indicating there may be an electrolyte disturbance or an element of renal failure;
- 12-lead ECG: looking for any rhythm disturbance as a cause for syncope;

- dipstick urine: collected as part of a septic work-up;
- CXR: looking for any signs of consolidation, as she is tachycardic and febrile.

The ECG has been obtained by nursing staff (see Fig. 3.1).

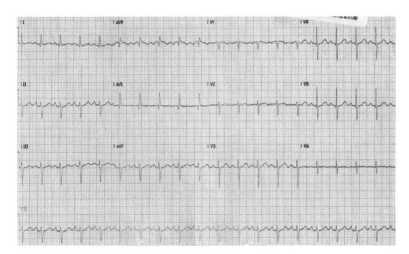

Figure 3.1 First ECG

Given that Mrs Jennings is dehydrated with postural hypotension, you commence intravenous rehydration with 0.9% normal saline at a rate of 1 litre over 2 hours. You decide to see another patient in the department while she is being rehydrated and waiting for the results of the investigations to come back.

11:10 hours

Some of the investigations are available for review (see Table 3.1).

Table 3.1 Pathology results

Assay	Result
Full blood count:	
Hb	142 g/L
WCC	14.5/nL
Neutrophils	12.2/nL
Platelets	303/nL
Urine:	Trace leucocytes

Her CXR has been performed (see Fig. 3.2).

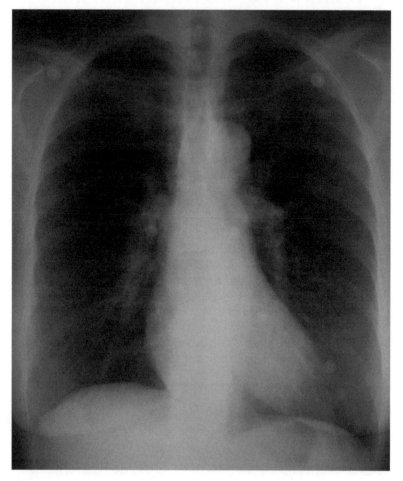

Figure 3.2 Chest X-ray

Clinical question 4

Review the results above.

(a) Do they help you in making a diagnosis?

(b) How will you proceed from here?

11:25 hours

After initial rehydration, Mrs Jennings feels somewhat better. However, you feel that it may take a little longer for the true situation to become clear, so you have little choice but to admit the patient for supportive care and observation. You feel that she has been hit hard by non-specific viral infection (it *is* influenza season and the hospital has been full of people with similar problems) so you arrange admission under the care of a medical unit. Mrs Jennings waits on a trolley for review and for an inpatient bed to become available.

16:45 hours

You're nearing the end of your shift when a member of the nursing staff calls the consultant emergency physician to see your patient urgently. You rush to the bedside to see what is happening.

Mrs Jennings is seriously ill. In fact, she looks like she is about to die. She is struggling to breathe, but despite taking large breaths she is still desperately breathless with a respiratory rate of 60 breaths per minute.

She is conscious but able to talk only in short, panting phrases. She is diaphoretic and looks 'blotchy' and 'mottled'. Her vital signs are:

- PR: 110 bpm
- temperature: 37.5°C
- BP: 140/100 mmHg
- SpO$_2$: 85% while breathing 15 L/min O$_2$

The consultant quickly examines her:

'Hmmm, normal chest examination, jugular venous pressure not seen, heart sounds dual, trachea midline, normal air entry with no added breath sounds ... this could only be one of a couple of things ...'

Clinical question 5

(a) What are the possibilities?
(b) What can you do about them?
(c) Describe what you will do regardless of what the diagnosis is.

Clinical comment

This is a serious situation that has occurred suddenly and catastrophically—what could possibly cause such a rapid deterioration? Regardless of the cause, resuscitation commences with oxygen and intravenous fluids. Something has put her into a state of shock. What are the diagnoses to consider?

Massive pulmonary embolism

This is supported by the sudden onset, and the fact that the chest sounds are normal and the patient is shocked: this is the classic 'obstructive' shock.

Pericardial tamponade

The pericardial sac could have reached a critical volume, impeding the ventricles' ability to fill and pump—one cause of obstructive shock. Hypotension would be expected. A pericardiocentesis could be performed if the suspicion is strong; alternatively, a less invasive approach could be to perform a bedside ultrasound scan and assess the pericardium. This could be done in seconds at the bedside.

Tension pneumothorax

It could present like this, but, against the diagnosis, the trachea is midline, and air entry is equal (though this is notoriously difficult to assess in a busy, noisy Emergency Department). The CXR showed no radiological features of a pneumothorax.

If tension pneumothorax is suspected, the treatment is to perform emergent pleurocentesis with a 14FG intravenous cannula inserted in the mid-clavicular line in the second intercostal space. If you're not sure which side is under tension you should perform the procedure on both left and right sides.

Physiology comment

A pulmonary embolism occurs most commonly when a blood clot passes from a deep vein in the lower limb through the right side of the heart and lodges in the main pulmonary artery or one of its sub-branches. Obstruction of pulmonary vessels by thromboemboli or tumour metastasis can lead to a reduction in the cross-sectional area of the pulmonary bed. If the reduction in area is large enough a sudden obstructive shock state occurs, with tachycardia, hypotension, shortness of breath, cyanosis and stupor. If the functional area of the pulmonary capillaries is not regained death can ensue in a matter of minutes.

16:55 hours

While the consultant explains to the patient and her husband what is unfolding, some bedside investigations are rapidly obtained: ABG, mobile CXR and ECG. The results are shown in Table 3.2, Figure 3.3 and Figure 3.4.

Table 3.2 Arterial blood gas results

FIO_2	0.8
pH	7.42
$PaCO_2$	26 mmHg
PaO_2	50 mmHg
HCO_3^-	19 mmol/L
BE	− 6

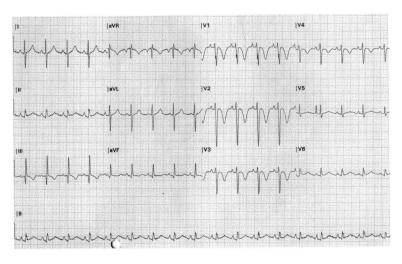

Figure 3.3 Second ECG

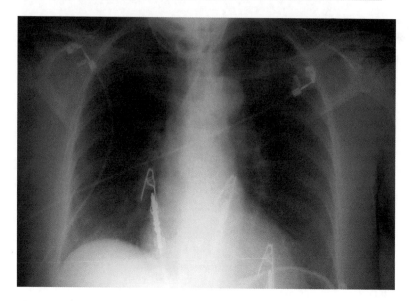

Figure 3.4 Second chest X-ray

 Clinical comment

Importantly, other diagnoses are ruled out: namely, tension pneumothorax, and acute myocardial ischaemia with cardiogenic shock:

- ECG: Sinus tachycardia with a 'S1Q3T3' pattern and signs of right heart strain. This is strongly suggestive of pulmonary embolism, but it should be noted that these classic findings are found in fewer of 20% of patients with pulmonary embolism.
- CXR: There may be reduced vascularity on the right lung: the so-called 'Westermark' sign. However, changes on plain X-rays are rarely seen in PE. The main purpose of chest radiography in this setting is to exclude alternative diagnoses.
- ABG: There is a large $P(A-a)O_2$ gradient, and a compensated metabolic acidosis. This doesn't affect management, but it does support the diagnosis. This is especially important given that the proposed therapy (thrombolysis) is potentially deadly itself and there is actually no Level 1 evidence supporting its efficacy in this setting.

These findings, combined with the dramatic clinical picture, are suggestive of a massive PE.

Physiology comment

A pulmonary embolism leads to a mismatch between alveolar ventilation and pulmonary blood flow (V/Q). Matching of ventilation to perfusion is critically important for effective gas exchange. Although there are regional differences in the V/Q ratio, the average for a healthy lung is approximately 0.8. In severe PE the V/Q approaches infinity; that is, extensive areas of the lung are ventilated, but not perfused. Virtually no gas exchange is possible in these regions and alveolar gas will have a similar composition to inspired air. A useful measure of ventilation–perfusion inequality is the alveolar–arterial PO_2 difference ($P(A\text{-}a)O_2$), which is obtained by subtracting the measured arterial PO_2 from a calculated alveolar value. A normal physiological shunt causes PaO_2 to be 5 to 15 mmHg below the alveolar value. A defining characteristic of V/Q mismatches is that they widen the $P(A\text{-}a)O_2$ gradient. The wider the $P(A\text{-}a)O_2$ gradient, the greater the severity of the V/Q mismatch.

Clinical question 6

(a) Are these investigations helpful?
(b) How do they affect your management right now?
(c) How will you explain to the patient what is going on?
(d) What information do you need before you administer further treatment?

17:00 hours

The results are reviewed and explained to the patient:

'Mrs Jennings, I realise you're feeling pretty awful, and this is due to a massive blood clot which has lodged in your lungs. All the investigations support it and I've ruled out other things that could make you feel this way. Our only option is to act quickly and give you a drug, which will dissolve that clot. It's potentially dangerous as you could bleed from other parts of your body, such as your brain. However, the risks of doing nothing are greater than the risks of giving you the drug, so I think we'd better proceed. What do you think?'

Mrs Jennings gasps her reply: 'Do whatever's best, Doctor ...'

Clinical question 7

What are the indications and contraindication of thrombolysis?

With the limited and rapid verbal consent, thrombolytic therapy is administered.

17:15 hours

Within 15 minutes Mrs Jennings is feeling much better: she is breathing much more easily, her pulse rate is settling and her perfusion is markedly improved. A heparin infusion is commenced. Now that she is stable, she is sent for a more definitive investigation to confirm the diagnosis.

Clinical question 8

(a) What imaging modalities are available for the diagnosis of PE?
(b) What role do blood tests such as the D-dimer play in this circumstance?

She is sent for a CTPA, which shows bilateral pulmonary emboli in the lower lobe segmental arteries.

18:15 hours

She is admitted to the CCU for observation and further investigation.

Clinical question 9

It is not enough to just diagnose a PE—we must also consider what has caused it in the first place.

(a) What are the causes of venous thrombosis and emboli?
(b) How can they be diagnosed?

Epilogue

A follow-up CT scan of the abdomen and pelvis revealed a large mass abutting Mrs Jennings' uterus and displacing her rectum. The pelvic veins were the most likely source of the emboli. The mass was subsequently removed at operation and found to be a benign tumour.

Clinical summary

Most emergency texts state: 'The diagnosis of pulmonary embolism should be considered in all patients with unexplained hypotension, syncope or hypoxaemic respiratory failure ...' However, as was observed with this patient, the clinical features can be ambiguous and it can be a difficult condition to diagnose. The following summary is provided to stimulate further discussion.

Pulmonary emboli

Pulmonary emboli present diagnostic and management challenges, and the following pointers place the condition in context:
- Pulmonary emboli account for up to 10–15% of in-hospital deaths.
- Pulmonary emboli have a high mortality rate.
- In one series, PE was not clinically considered in up to 70% of PEs diagnosed at autopsy.
- 70% have proximal deep vein thrombosis.
- One or more risk factors are present in 80–90% of diagnosed PEs.

There are many issues to consider in this patient, and they can be broadly divided into diagnosis and management.

Diagnosis

How do you actually diagnose PE in this patient before it becomes life-threatening? In retrospect, PE seems an obvious diagnosis. There were a number of important findings to consider, such as the unexplained tachycardia and the postural blood pressure drop. Would standard therapy such as anticoagulation with subcutaneous low molecular weight heparin a few hours earlier have prevented the life-threatening deterioration later in the day? It seems unlikely, but we will never know.

Would a D-dimer blood test have assisted diagnosis? In retrospect it may have led to an earlier diagnosis. In general it is a test that should be used and interpreted with caution, depending upon the patient group. In patients where there is a high level of suspicion for the diagnosis of PE a negative result may not rule out the diagnosis, and further investigations should be performed. Computer tomography pulmonary angiogram has largely replaced ventilation/perfusion scanning for this purpose, but as is the case with most interventions and investigations, approaches vary on availability of staff and equipment in different institutions.

How do you rapidly diagnose the condition once the patient has deteriorated? Decisions often have to be made in emergency situations before the complete information is available. In this circumstance the diagnosis was made on the basis of a combination of the rapid exclusion of alternative diagnoses and clinical probability.

Management

Thrombolysis for pulmonary emboli is a controversial topic. Level 1 evidence with well-defined indications exists for thrombolytic therapy in acute myocardial infarction. Thrombolysis for PE, however, is an evolving indication in that Level 1 evidence for this intervention is not yet available, but the therapy is becoming accepted practice in many institutions. Evidence-based medicine would not look kindly on this, but intuitively it makes sense. In general, the rationale to administer thrombolytic therapy is based upon clinical judgment in the presence of PE with acute right heart strain. In general, lysis is offered for massive PE (where the patient has arrested) and sub-massive PE (as in this circumstance, where there is right heart strain and the patient is about to arrest). In these circumstances it can be argued that the benefits of therapy outweigh the risks. In most pulmonary emboli, where there is little compromise at the time of diagnosis, the risks of therapy outweigh the benefits and anticoagulation alone is adequate.

References and further reading

1 Calder, K.K., Herbert, M., Henderson, S.O. The mortality of untreated pulmonary embolism in emergency department patients. Ann Emerg Med 2005 Mar; 45(3): 302–10.
2 Garg, K., Macey, L. Helical CT scanning in the diagnosis of pulmonary embolism. Respiration 2003 May–Jun; 70(3): 231–7.
3 Goldhaber, S.Z., Elliott, C.G. Acute pulmonary embolism: Part I Epidemiology, pathophysiology, and diagnosis. Circulation 2003; 108: 2726–9.
4 Goldhaber, S.Z., Elliott, C.G. Acute pulmonary embolism: Part II Risk stratification, treatment, and prevention. Circulation 2003; 108: 2834–8.
5 Konstantinides, S., Geibel, A., Heusel, G. et al. Heparin plus alteplase compared with heparin alone in patients with submassive pulmonary embolism. N Engl J Med 2002 Oct 10; 347(15): 1143–50.

Review

Level 1: Content knowledge

1 The majority of pulmonary emboli originate from thrombi in the:
   A Lungs
   B Right heart
   C Left heart
   D Leg and pelvic veins
   E Pulmonary veins

2 Which of the following may cause a poor orthostatic response?
   A Reduced ability of the autonomic nervous system to increase heart rate and stroke volume and therefore cardiac output
   B Reduced ability of the autonomic nervous system to increase TPR
   C Reduced total blood volume
   D Maldistribution of blood volume
   E All of the above

3 The alveolar–arterial PO_2 difference $P(A\text{-}a)O_2$ is typically:
   A 0–5 mmHg
   B 5–15 mmHg
   C 15–25 mmHg
   D 25–35 mmHg

Level 2: Clinical applications

1 Which is the most common ECG finding in patients with pulmonary embolism?
   A Right heart strain
   B S1-Q3-T3 pattern
   C ST segment depression in the lateral leads
   D Sinus tachycardia
   E Atrial fibrillation

2 Which of the following is *not* a risk factor for thromboembolic disease?
   A Obesity
   B Prolonged immobilisation
   C Cigarette smoking
   D Neoplastic disease
   E All of the above are risk factors

3 Which of the following investigations is the *least* helpful in assessing this scenario?

A 32-year-old woman presents with the sudden onset of breathlessness and sharp left sided chest pain 2 weeks after an arthroscopy. She is tachycardic. She is on the contraceptive pill and is not pregnant.

A Chest radiography
B D-dimer
C 12-lead ECG
D CT pulmonary angiogram
E Pulse oximetry

Level 3: Topics for further discussion

1 Compare and contrast the different diagnostic aids for diagnosing pulmonary embolism.
2 Discuss the different therapies available for pulmonary embolism and the evidence behind them.

Case 4
Christopher had never felt this sick before ...

This 25-year-old man presents with a history of chest pain and breathlessness, presenting the team in the Emergency Department with a range of possible diagnoses. It's critical to make the right diagnosis quickly—failure to do so could have dire consequences. Nevertheless, initial therapy is directed to restoring perfusion to vital organs.

Timeline summary

10:07	Arrives in the Emergency Department.
10:11	Combined nursing and medical assessment begins; arterial blood gas (ABG) taken and oxygen applied.
10:14	Directed history obtained; vital signs obtained.
10:17	Physical examination performed and intravenous access obtained; venous blood collected simultaneously.
10:19	Intravenous fluid commenced; antibiotics administered.
10:24	Mobile chest X-ray (CXR) available for viewing on the viewing box; computer tomography pulmonary angiogram (CTPA) arranged; intensive care unit (ICU) warned of likely admission.
10:30–11:00	Continued fluid and oxygen therapy with good response.
11:05	Sent for CTPA; blood results available.
11:25	CTPA results phoned through to the Emergency Department.
13:00	Inpatient bed available; patient transferred to ICU.

Learning objectives

Physiological

- Outline how respiratory alkalosis can develop in pneumonia.
- Describe the structural and functional changes to lung tissue associated with pneumonia.
- Understand how these structural and functional changes are linked to the clinical signs of the disease.

Clinical

- Understand the different ways that patients with sepsis may present to hospital.
- Know the appropriate investigations to utilise when assessing the patient with suspected thromboembolic disease.
- Be able to interpret the ABG results in a clinical setting.

Context

Christopher had never been this sick before. Nearly 26 years old, he worked hard and had literally never had a sick day in his life. But today was more than 'just the flu'. He had been woken from his sleep just after midnight with a terrible pain in the right side of his chest and feeling hot. It was sharp, he could hardly breathe, and he was coughing a lot. To make matters worse there had been blood in his phlegm on a couple of occasions. Put simply, he felt awful.

However, with his typical determination and down-to-earth approach to life, he hoped it would all go away, and it was only at 10:00 a.m. that his girlfriend finally convinced him that something was wrong and that he should seek urgent medical attention. She bundled him into the car and shortly after he arrived at the Emergency Department at the local hospital. He was conscious on arrival and was triaged 'category 2', and was wheeled through to a monitored area.

10:07 hours

Christopher arrives in the Emergency Department.

Clinical question 1

(a) What would be your immediate actions upon meeting Christopher?

(b) Discuss how you would start assessing and managing him.

10:11 hours

Christopher is met by a member of the nursing staff who begins her assessment and applies monitoring equipment. A member of the medical staff is present as well, and obtains an arterial blood sample just before administering high-flow oxygen therapy.

10:14 hours

The medical staff member rapidly obtains Christopher's history, and additionally learns that he had some episodes of extreme shivering overnight. He denied any drug use or recent travel. However, Christopher is finding it hard to speak because of his extreme breathlessness. The doctor feels Christopher's radial pulse, and notes that it is rapid and feeble. He listens to his chest and hears coarse crackles and a friction rub over his right lung.

Christopher's vital signs are as follows:

- PR: 140 bpm
- RR: 40 breaths/min
- BP: 80/– mmHg
- SpO_2: 83% on room air; 98% on 15 L/min of O_2 via non-rebreathing bag
- temperature: 37.3°C

Clinical question 2

(a) What diagnoses are going through your mind at this early stage?

(b) What will be your management at this time?

(c) What clinical findings would you be specifically looking for?

Clinical comment

Christopher appears to be seriously ill. This young man, who is usually in excellent health, is now unwell with markedly abnormal vital signs.

Possible diagnoses include pulmonary embolism, pneumothorax, pericarditis with tamponade, and pneumonia. Initial clinical examination and assessment should be directed towards identifying these important diagnoses.

Initial therapy would be supportive regardless of the cause: oxygen, intravenous access and fluid resuscitation. These interventions occur regardless of the ultimate diagnosis and are a practical application of the dictum: 'Assessment and management occur in parallel.'

10:17 hours

The doctor completes the physical examination on Christopher and notes the following:

- Trachea is central.
- Jugular venous pressure (JVP) is not clinically elevated.
- Heart sounds are clearly heard.
- Calves are non-tender and not swollen.

Clinical comment

These findings are rapidly elicited and are of critical importance. In a few seconds the diagnoses of tension pneumothorax (trachea midline), pericardial tamponade (Beck's triad, although unreliable for diagnosis, is not present) and pulmonary embolism (no source of thrombus immediately apparent) have been considered.

These important diagnoses have not been ruled out by the absence of any positive signs, but their presence becomes less likely.

Intravenous access is obtained and blood is collected for laboratory testing. A mobile CXR is urgently arranged. Meanwhile, the results of the ABG that was taken on room air upon Christopher's arrival only a few short minutes ago are available (see Table 4.1).

Table 4.1 Arterial blood gas results

FIO_2	0.21
pH	7.46
$PaCO_2$	28.7 mmHg
PaO_2	45.4 mmHg
HCO_3^-	19.5 mmol/L

Clinical question 3

(a) Interpret the ABG result.

(b) What blood tests would you request? Justify each request and discuss how it will assist in your diagnosis and management.

Physiology comment

The arterial blood gas results indicate a respiratory alkalosis (pH > 7.45; low $PaCO_2$) secondary to hypoxaemia (low PaO_2). A low PaO_2 in the blood is sensed by chemoreceptors, which stimulate an increase in the rate and depth of breathing via the respiratory centre. The resulting loss of carbon dioxide leads to the respiratory alkalosis. The blood gas results indicate that some compensation has occurred, as the bicarbonate is lower than normal. In this case (see later diagnosis) the underlying hypoxaemia is caused by V/Q mismatching (decreased alveolar ventilation is due to consolidation of acini) and diffusion impairment (caused by damage to the alveolar/capillary membrane).

Clinical comment

The ABG can be interpreted as follows:

- pH: mild alkalaemia;
- $PaCO_2$: low;
- PaO_2: low;
- HCO_3^-: low.

Interpretation: Type 1 respiratory failure with a compensated metabolic acidosis and a respiratory alkalosis.

This suggests that Christopher is quite unwell and is struggling to maintain his blood oxygen levels. If someone is hypoxaemic it is accepted practice that the hypoxaemia be treated immediately; that is, do not withhold oxygen just so that staff can take a blood test. However, the test was taken rapidly as oxygen was being applied. The fact that the pH is in the alkalotic range does not mean the acidosis is not present—Christopher is just compensating well at this stage. He is trying to increase the partial pressure of oxygen in his alveoli by hyperventilating.

The following pathology tests are requested:

- full blood count (FBC)—to assess the inflammatory response;
- urea and electrolytes (U & E's)—to assess renal function and electrolyte balance;
- blood cultures—to provide a microbiological diagnosis.

10:19 hours

Now that vascular access has been obtained, intravenous fluids are commenced. Given his hypotension and tachycardia, 1 litre of 0.9% normal saline is commenced as a bolus. Given that a severe community-acquired pneumonia producing sepsis is considered, antibiotics are rapidly administered: 1.2 g of intravenous penicillin and 150 mg of oral roxithromycin.

Clinical question 4

Discuss the evidence for the choice of antibiotics in this circumstance.

10:24 hours

The radiographer arrives and takes a mobile chest X-ray (see Figure 4.1).

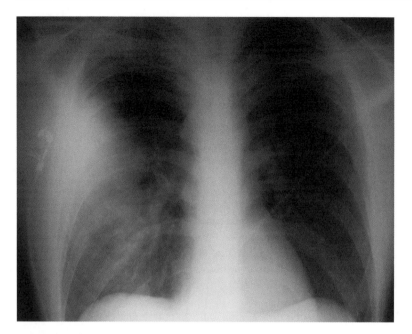

Figure 4.1 Chest X-ray

Clinical question 5

(a) Describe the CXR.
(b) Does this rule in or rule out any particular diagnosis?

The doctor looks at the CXR and carefully considers the situation.

'Hmmm ... he's shocked, he's got wedge-shaped consolidation, and it all came on suddenly. He swears he was perfectly well when he went to bed. I thought he'd have community-acquired pneumonia, but this raises the possibility of a pulmonary embolus.'

10:30–11:00 hours

Meanwhile, his blood pressure has risen to 110/60 mmHg and his pulse has reduced to 110 bpm after 1 litre of saline. He is feeling marginally better, but is still finding it hard to breathe.

Clinical question 6

(a) What will you do now? List the possible outcomes at this stage.
(b) What diagnostic aids are available to diagnose pulmonary embolism (PE)?
(c) What would be your pre-test probability of a PE? Discuss why this is important.

Clinical comment

The CXR shows wedge-shaped consolidation in the right lung. This could be consistent with pneumonia, but importantly raises the possibility of pulmonary embolism. Resuscitation with oxygen and intravenous fluid must continue, regardless of the cause. However, making a timely and correct diagnosis is important because of the range of different therapies available.

Calculating the clinical probability of pulmonary embolism is important, as all investigations have limitations and results cannot be relied upon in isolation. This principle applies especially to ventilation/perfusion scanning (where a significant proportion of patients with a 'low probability' scan have proven thromboembolic disease), but applies to all investigations. Simply put, investigations test hypotheses and must be interpreted in light of clinical findings and individual circumstances.

A CTPA is organised. Meanwhile, the first pathology results become available on the computer (see Table 4.2).

Table 4.2 Pathology results

Test	Result	Normal range
FBC:		
Hb	143	130–175 g/L
WCC	33.9	3.5–11.0/nL
Neutrophils	30.6	1.5–7.5/nL
Platelets	226	160–420/nL
Biochemistry:		
Na⁺	134	135–145 mmol/L
K⁺	3.5	3.5–5.0 mmol/L
Urea	5.0	2.7–7.8 mmol/L
Creatinine	91	60–115 mmol/L

Clinical question 7

(a) Comment upon and interpret these blood tests.
(b) How do they affect your management at this stage?

His condition remains unchanged during the CTPA scan as the images come through (see Fig. 4.2).

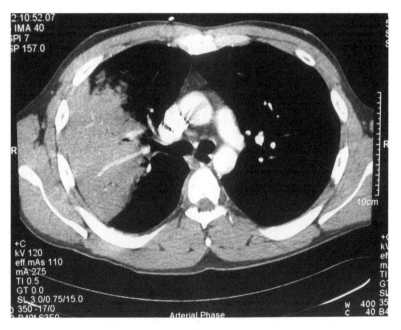

Figure 4.2 Computer tomography pulmonary angiogram

11:25 hours

The radiologist rings through the results to the treating doctor:

> 'There is extensive airspace opacification of the right upper and middle lobes with air bronchogram consistent with infective consolidation. There are blood vessels seen running through these areas of consolidation.
>
> 'There is satisfactory contrast enhancement of the pulmonary trunk and the segmental pulmonary arteries. No filling defects are seen to suggest the presence of pulmonary emboli.

'Conclusion: Extensive consolidation of the right upper and middle lobes. No evidence of pulmonary embolism.'

Clinical question 8

(a) Can you now rule out PE as the cause?

(b) What is the most likely aetiology of his pneumonia? Consider your local epidemiology as you discuss this.

13:00 hours

Given the severity of his presenting symptoms and signs, the emergency consultant had arranged for Christopher to be admitted to hospital for continuing care.

Epilogue

Christopher steadily improved over the next 24 hours, with his vital signs improving and his CXR showing progressive resolution of the consolidation in the right upper and middle lobes. The blood cultures signalled positive after 24 hours, and the results were soon available (Table 4.3).

Table 4.3 Blood culture results

Aerobic bottle:	*Positive* after 1 day's incubation
Culture	
Organism:	1. *Streptococcus pneumoniae*
Sensitivities: 1	Penicillin S

The final diagnosis was *Streptococcus pneumoniae* (community-acquired pneumonia). He had scored less than 90 on the Pneumonia Severity Index (PSI), thereby placing him in an intermediate risk category. Christopher steadily improved and was discharged home after a total of 4 days in hospital.

Physiology comment

Pneumonia is inflammation of the lungs caused by bacteria, viruses or chemical compounds. The case presentation is typical of pneumococci, staphylococci or bacilli in that it had a sudden onset and was associated with chills, high fever, chest pain and production of bloody sputum. In healthy individuals it is possible for pathogens entering the lungs to overwhelm the body's normal defences, but infection usually occurs in immune-compromised individuals.

The typical progression of a pneumonia case can be explained by understanding the underlying physiology. In the above case aspiration of the *Streptococcus pneumoniae* led to a sequence of structural and functional changes to the lung tissue that explain the signs of the disease. Understanding these changes also informs the treatment regime that is adopted in the case.

The sequences of events that are linked to the aspiration of the bacteria are outlined in the diagram below.

The clinical manifestations in pneumonia (listed below) can be explained when the sequence of events is understood.

- fever and leukocytosis (> 10 000 per mm^3)—systemic signs of infection;
- dyspnoea and tachypnoea—increased work of breathing;
- bloody or foul smelling sputum;

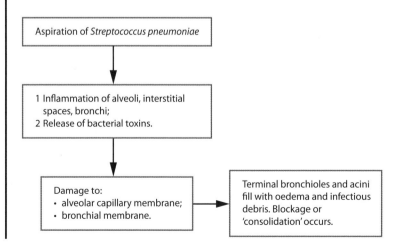

Aspiration of *Streptococcus pneumoniae*

1 Inflammation of alveoli, interstitial spaces, bronchi;
2 Release of bacterial toxins.

Damage to:
- alveolar capillary membrane;
- bronchial membrane.

Terminal bronchioles and acini fill with oedema and infectious debris. Blockage or 'consolidation' occurs.

- rhonchi (coarse rattling sounds due to fluid movement in larger airways) and crackles (finer sounds associated with the opening and closing of alveoli);
- consolidated areas may have no breath sounds;
- atelectasis and consolidations may be present on the chest X-ray;
- lung inflammation is associated with dull chest pain.

Clinical summary

This patient appeared seriously ill and required urgent and effective therapy. Risk stratification can be performed by using various clinical scoring systems, and can assist with disposition. Despite his dramatic appearance, validated scoring systems such as the PSI suggest that he was at a relatively low risk of suffering an adverse outcome. Pneumonia has a high mortality in elderly and immunocompromised patients, and those with co-morbidities.

The blood tests revealed a significant inflammatory response, consistent with an infective cause. It must be remembered that a raised white cell count can occur in a number of situations other than infection, and therefore the result did not alter management in this patient's case.

Basic life support measures of a primary survey are applicable in this instance, and the supportive care he received would be appropriate regardless of the aetiology. Pneumonia can develop rapidly, but it would be unwise to disregard pulmonary embolism as a possible cause. Pulmonary embolism can be diagnosed with a number of different modalities, and they vary from hospital to hospital, depending upon the services and expertise available. These include CTPA, ventilation/perfusion scanning, and Doppler ultrasound. There is a limited role for the use of blood tests such as D-dimers in the diagnosis of thromboembolic disease—when there is a high clinical suspicion for the disease the D-dimer test loses significance, and therefore should not be used as an aid to diagnosis in high-risk patients. In this circumstance an alternative diagnosis was made using CT scanning, and pulmonary embolism could then be discounted. This is the benefit of CTPA in this instance: alternative conditions can be diagnosed.

Pneumococcus remains the most common cause of community-acquired pneumonia in Australia and antimicrobial therapy should be directed against this pathogen. Penicillin remains the antibiotic of choice, and macrolide antibiotics are recommended to cover against atypical organisms such as *Mycoplasma*. Clinicians must be careful when using antibiotics and refer to evidence-based guidelines to reduce inappropriate antibiotic usage, which can contribute to the growing worldwide problem of resistance.

It could be said that this patient was suffering from the early stages of septic shock: he certainly had abnormal vital signs suggesting impaired perfusion of his organs. However, he had a normal mental state, suggesting either adequate compensation or that he had systemic inflammatory response syndrome (SIRS; a systemic inflammatory response to a variety of severe clinical insults), i.e. a 'pre-sepsis' state. Either way, early recognition of the severity of his condition and early aggressive therapy is important to reduce mortality.

SIRS is characterised by two or more of the following conditions:

- temperature higher than 38°C or lower than 36°C;
- heart rate higher than 90 bpm;
- respiratory rate higher than 20 breaths/min or $PaCO_2$ lower than 32 mmHg;
- white blood cell counts higher than 12 000 cells/mm^3 or lower than 4000 cells/mm^3, or the presence of more than 10% immature neutrophils ('band cells').

References and further reading

1 *British Thoracic Society Guidelines for the Management of Community Acquired Pneumonia in Adults*—2004 update. http://www.brit-thoracic.org.uk/docs/MACAPrevisedApr04.pdf
2 Fine, M.J., Auble,T.E., Yealy, D.M. et al. A prediction rule to identify low-risk patients with community-acquired pneumonia. N Engl J Med 1997; 336: 243–50.
3 Johnson, P.D.R., Irving, L.B. and Turnidge, J.D. MJA practice essentials—infectious diseases: Community-acquired pneumonia. MJA 2002; 176: 341–7. http://www.mja.com.au/public/issues/176_07_010402/joh10289_fm.html
4 Lim, W.S., van der Eerden, M.M., Laing, R., Boersma, W.G., Karalus, N., Town, G.I., Lewis, S.A., Macfarlane, J.T. Defining community acquired pneumonia severity on presentation to hospital: an international derivation and validation study. Thorax 2003; 58:377–82. http://thorax.bmjjournals.com/cgi/content/full/58/5/377

Review

Level 1: Content knowledge

1 The typical presentation of pneumococci-, staphylococci- or bacilli-induced pneumonia includes all of the following *except*:
   A Chills
   B High fever
   C Abdominal pain
   D Production of bloody sputum
2 The hypoxaemia associated with pneumonia is caused by:
   A Decreased pulmonary perfusion
   B Anaemia
   C V/Q mismatching and diffusion impairment
   D Global hypoventilation
3 $PaCO_2$ is often low initially in pneumonia because:
   A The individual has impaired diffusing capacity.
   B The individual hyperventilates to compensate for the low PaO_2.
   C The alveoli of the individual become consolidated.
   D The individual hypoventilates to compensate for the low PaO_2.

Level 2: Clinical applications

1 A 45-year-old male with no past medical history is diagnosed with community-acquired pneumonia. Which of the following organisms is the most likely pathogen?
   A *Mycoplasma pneumoniae*
   B *Haemophilus influenzae*
   C *Streptococcus pneumoniae*
   D *Pseudomonas aeruginosa*
   E *Staphylococcus aureus*
2 Match the following pathogens with the most appropriate antimicrobial therapy:
   A *Mycoplasma pneumoniae*
   B *Haemophilus influenzae*
   C *Streptococcus pneumoniae*
   D *Pseudomonas aeruginosa*
   E *Staphylococcus aureus*
   　(i) Benzyl penicillin
   　(ii) Macrolide antibiotic (such as roxithromycin)
   　(iii) Flucloxacillin
   　(iv) Ceftazidime
   　(v) Amoxycillin/clavulanic acid

3 Which of the following chest X-ray findings support a diagnosis of *Streptococcus* pneumonia?

   A Consolidation in the left lower lobe

   B Kerley B lines in the left and right lower lobes

   C Air space destruction in both lobes

   D Abscess formation with air-fluid levels in the right upper lobe

   E Upper lobe vascular redistribution

Level 3: Topics for further discussion

1 Discuss the use of various scoring systems and guidelines that can be used to guide disposition and antimicrobial therapy.

2 Describe your understanding of the central role of pathology laboratories and public health staff in guiding empirical therapy in your region.

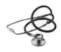

Case 5
Frank ran into trouble out on the water ...

This 67-year-old male spends most days out on the water, fishing from his powerboat. But today something goes terribly wrong, and he is brought to the Emergency Department after being rescued by the water police. He is drowsy and can give no history—now it is up to you to both assess and manage him appropriately.

Timeline summary

09:10	Crew on a fishing boat report a small cabin cruiser behaving erratically and notify the water police. The fishing boat is unable to safely approach or board the vessel.
10:23	Water police officers and a paramedic board vessel and find an elderly male unconscious inside an enclosed cabin; they call the ambulance and arrange a rendezvous.
11:15	Water police vessel arrives at jetty; the male patient is handed over to care of paramedics; oxygen is administered.
11:30	Patient arrives at hospital; semi-conscious; triaged category 1; medical and nursing team standing by to begin treatment.
11:30–12:25	Resuscitation and investigations: a 12-lead electrocardiogram (ECG) and arterial blood gas (ABG) are taken.
12:45	Transfer to definitive therapy.

Learning objectives

Physiological

- Understand the role of haemoglobin in delivering sufficient oxygen to the tissues.
- Describe Dalton's law regarding partial pressures of gases in a mixture.
- Describe how pressure differences determine net diffusion of gases through a liquid.
- Understand the difference between haemoglobin saturation and oxygen content of the blood.
- Be able to identify the properties of the oxyhaemoglobin dissociation curve that are relevant to carbon monoxide poisoning.
- Understand the physiological basis of carbon monoxide toxicity.
- Be able to identify and explain the physiological basis of the signs and symptoms associated with carbon monoxide poisoning.
- Describe the physiological basis of carbon monoxide poisoning treatment.

Clinical

- Understand the principles of assessing and managing the patient with a reduced conscious state.
- Describe the causes of unconsciousness in humans.
- Appreciate how different branches of the emergency services work together in a coordinated manner to provide optimal pre-hospital patient care.
- Be able to utilise appropriate investigations in the assessment of the patient with a reduced conscious state.
- Be able to recognise environmental causes of a decreased state of consciousness.
- Recognise the possibility of carbon monoxide poisoning as a cause for unconsciousness and the indications for hyperbaric oxygen therapy.

Context

Frank enjoyed fishing; in fact, now that he was retired, he tried to get out onto the water as often as he could. He had bought an old but seaworthy cabin cruiser with his superannuation payout and, despite the occasional bit of engine trouble (which he was usually able to repair himself), he would check the weather almost every morning and go fishing off the coast of southern Tasmania. Today was like any other day, and by 9:00 a.m. in the morning he was in the open sea.

09:10 hours

The crew of a fishing trawler heading out to sea notice a small vessel motoring around in circles. They can see someone slumped inside the enclosed cabin. Deciding it is too unsafe to get too close because of the increasing ocean swell, they radio the water police and request help. In the meantime they keep a close eye on the boat and prepare themselves to render assistance if required. The police immediately dispatch a boat with a paramedic onboard.

10:23 hours

The police vessel reaches the boat and the crew are able to board it. They find an elderly male inside the cabin, unconscious but breathing. They secure the boat and proceed to return to port with the paramedic administering oxygen and nursing him in the coma position. The treating paramedic requests that his communications centre notify the receiving hospital of the current status of the patient and their expected time of arrival.

11:15 hours

The police return to port; the emergency services communication centres had been coordinating the operation and an ambulance is waiting. The paramedic reports that the patient has improved slightly and that he now has a GCS of 12. The patient is loaded into the back of the ambulance and they proceed to the hospital.

11:30 hours

The emergency physician on duty had been aware of the unfolding situation since 9:30 a.m. A team had been assembled and is waiting for the patient's arrival.

Clinical question 1

(a) What sort of information would you require from the treating paramedic?

(b) Describe how you would prepare for this patient's arrival.

(c) Discuss your differential diagnoses.

The patient is wheeled in on a trolley and the paramedic begins his handover to the emergency physician:

'He was unconscious but breathing when I first saw him: GCS 6 (E1 V2 M3), PR 110, BP 100/60, RR 22. He was inside the cabin of his boat, with the engine still running. I placed him into the coma position and applied high-flow oxygen. His pupils were equal and as we proceeded to shore he steadily improved to where he is now. I placed an 18G cannula in his left wrist and commenced IV Hartmann's. He's had 500 mL over the last hour.'

Frank is quickly transferred to the hospital trolley. The emergency physician assumes the role of team leader and coordinates the assessment and management from the end of the bed as the team carries out its work.

The team applies the appropriate monitoring equipment and begins their assessment and management.

Clinical question 2

(a) Given the above information, list your management priorities.
(b) Is there any extra information you would like at this stage?

The following information becomes readily apparent as the team examines the patient:

- airway: patent
- breathing: rapid; RR 22 breaths/min
- SpO_2:   98% on 15 L O_2/min
- circulation: PR 80 bpm; BP 120/85 mmHg
- disability: GCS 12 (E3 V4 M5); pupils 4 mm and reactive

'No rashes, or signs of head trauma', reports the doctor at the airway.

'I've placed a 16G cannula into his right arm and I'm collecting blood', calls the second doctor.

'BSL 8.6', reports one of the nurses.

The consultant looks at the patient and turns to the resident.

'Could you take arterial blood sample for blood gas analysis right now?'

Turning back to the team, she continues:

'Let's take a 12-lead ECG and urgently send the bloods to pathology; could radiography come and take a chest X-ray and we may need to quickly transport him to radiology for a CT scan of his brain.'

Clinical comment

The assessment and management of the unconscious patient is a medical emergency. Treatment begins when the patient is first discovered, and is directed towards maintaining his airway and breathing until definitive support can be provided. Anyone can do basic first aid, and it can be life-saving. The cause is less important in the early stages—keeping the patient alive takes priority.

This patient was rescued by utilising multiple arms of the emergency services. A coordinated approach with well-defined lines of communication is essential, and is the hallmark of any emergency medical system. Although it is important for doctors to be aware of important conditions occurring in individuals, it is equally important for them to be aware of and take a leadership role in the emergency medical systems surrounding them. Different regions have differing systems requirements and designs, so it is essential that you be aware of what is in operation in your region.

There are a number of possible causes for an altered mental state. Sometimes the cause is immediately obvious, but in other cases a more rigorous history, examination and investigation is required. A well-known mnemonic to assist with diagnosis is 'AEIOU TIPS':

A	Alcohol and other toxins	**T**	Trauma
E	Endocrinopathy	**I**	Infection
	Encephalopathy	**P**	Psychogenic
	Electrolyte disturbances	**S**	Seizure
I	Insulin—diabetes		Syncope
O	Oxygen: hypoxia of any cause		Space-occupying lesion
	Opiates		
U	Uraemia including hypertension		

Assessment and management should be directed to considering these potential causes. Some causes may be rapidly excluded by a directed clinical examination (for example, signs of a head injury or a toxidrome); others may require a simple bedside test (such as a blood glucose level); or it may be necessary to perform a computer tomography (CT) scan of the brain (to identify an intracerebral bleed).

Regardless of the cause, assessment and management must occur in parallel. Life-saving therapy should not be delayed while a diagnosis is sought.

Clinical question 3

Given the above information, is a particular diagnosis becoming more likely?

The nurse performs an ECG and hands it to the team leader for review (see Fig. 5.1).

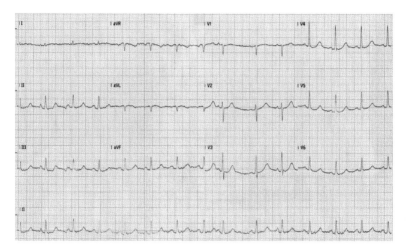

Figure 5.1 ECG

Clinical question 4

(a) Comment upon the ECG.
(b) How can an ECG assist you in determining the causes of a reduced conscious state?

The team continues its assessment and steadily the picture becomes clearer. The paramedic is still present.

The consultant turns to him. 'Tell me; was there an odour in the cabin?'

Before he can answer, the resident returns with the ABG results (see Table 5.1).

Table 5.1 Arterial blood gas results

FIO$_2$	1.0
Blood gas values:	
pH	7.386
PaCO$_2$	37.4 mmHg
PaO$_2$	314 mmHg
BE	−2.1 mmol/L
HCO$_3^-$	22.0 mmol/L
Oximetry values:	
Hb	132 g/L
SaO$_2$	99.6%
COHb	29.6%
Electrolyte values:	
K$^+$	3.6 mmol/L
Na$^+$	141 mmol/L
Metabolite values:	
Glu	7.9 mmol/L

Clinical question 5

(a) Describe the ABG results.
(b) What is the diagnosis?
(c) How did this situation occur?
(d) Does this exclude any other possible causes for his reduced conscious state?
(e) Discuss the treatment options.

The consultant looked at the carboxyhaemoglobin result:

'Looks like he's had a significant exposure to carbon monoxide; we'd better refer him to the hyperbaric oxygen unit. Keep looking for other causes, he might have collapsed and then been exposed to the fumes.'

Physiology comment

Gas pressures of individual gases and gas mixtures

The pressure that a gas exerts against a surface is due to the impact of the gas molecules that are striking the surface at any given time. The pressure a gas exerts is therefore directly related to the concentration of the gas molecules that are present. Dalton's law states that the total pressure of a gas mixture equals the sum of the pressures exerted by each component. The basis for this is that each gas component exerts the pressure (its partial pressure) that would be exerted if it alone occupied the total volume. The key point is that the difference in partial pressure between two sites determines the rate and direction of diffusion. For example, oxygen will normally diffuse from arterial blood to working skeletal tissue, as a large oxygen gradient normally exists.

Pressures of gases dissolved in liquid

It is a bit harder to visualise how a gas dissolved in the liquid phase can exert a pressure. Gases dissolved in water do in fact exert a pressure when the liquid comes into contact with a surface, much the same way they do in the gas phase. This is because the dissolved gas molecules have kinetic energy and are therefore continually moving within the liquid and when they collide with a surface they exert a pressure. For example, if blood is exposed to a gas whose oxygen partial pressure is such that there is no net oxygen exchange, then the partial pressure of oxygen (PO_2) in the blood is the same as that in the gas.

Gas transport

For normal cellular function oxygen has to be continually transported from the lungs to the tissues via the blood at a rate equal to the tissues' metabolic demand. A small amount of oxygen is carried in the plasma as dissolved oxygen, but most is transported in chemical combination with the carrier molecule haemoglobin (Hb). Haemoglobin consists of four polypeptide chains, each with an oxygen-carrying haem group. As the PO_2 in plasma increases, oxygen combines reversibly with haem forming oxyhaemoglobin. The greater the PO_2, the greater number of oxygen binding sites that are occupied by oxygen. The presence of Hb greatly increases the amount of oxygen that can be carried in the blood than is possible if transportation was reliant on the solubility of oxygen in plasma alone.

Haemoglobin saturation (%)

The Hb saturation is the percentage of haem binding sites that have been occupied by oxygen. It is important to understand that saturation does not tell us anything about the number of binding sites (that is, the Hb concentration) that are present, but only the percentage of the total available that have been occupied.

Oxygen content of the blood

This is the total amount of oxygen carried in the blood and is usually expressed as mL oxygen per 100 mL blood. This typically comprises 97% oxygen bound with Hb and 3% oxygen dissolved in plasma. Oxygen content depends not only on the amount of Hb present, but also the PO_2. Oxygen saturation on the other hand, for a given partial pressure of carbon dioxide (PCO_2), pH and temperature, depends solely on the PaO_2. An oxyhaemoglobin dissociation curve therefore cannot tell us how much oxygen is being carried unless the amount of Hb present is known.

Oxygen dissociation curve

The oxygen dissociation curve describes the combination of Hb with oxygen. When a molecule of oxygen binds with haem a conformational change occurs (an allosteric effect), increasing the affinity of the next binding site for oxygen. This explains in part the sigmoid shape of the oxyhaemoglobin dissociation curve. This relationship between PO_2 and percentage saturation is important as it facilitates offloading of oxygen from Hb at low partial pressures (blood flowing through the tissues) and facilitates the binding of oxygen with Hb at high partial pressures (blood flowing through the pulmonary capillaries).

A range of factors, including pH, PCO_2, temperature and 2,3-diphosphoglycerate levels, can alter the shape and position of the oxyhaemoglobin dissociation curve, therefore altering the percentage saturation of Hb at any given PO_2. Carbon monoxide binds to haem and shifts the curve to the left. This means that Hb that has carbon monoxide bound to it has a greater affinity for oxygen at any given partial pressure than it normally would have. This means that not only is the amount of oxygen delivered to the tissues reduced in carbon monoxide poisoning, but whatever oxygen is present is bound more tightly than normal, worsening tissue hypoxia.

Clinical comment

The carboxyhaemoglobin of 29.6% indicates a significant exposure to carbon monoxide. This may be accidental or intentional; keep in mind that carbon monoxide is a common method of committing suicide in Australia. This will require further consideration once Frank is back to good health and a complete history can be obtained. Carbon monoxide is produced by the incomplete combustion of hydrocarbons; therefore a faulty motor and/or inadequate ventilation is able to cause the condition. Carbon monoxide itself is odourless, but other substances associated with its production may create a noticeable smell, thus alerting clinicians to the diagnosis. It is in fact one of the most common causes of injury and death due to poisoning in the world.

Clinicians must remember that there are other potential causes for Frank's reduced level of consciousness which should still be considered. It is possible that Frank suffered a syncopal episode that resulted in him being unable to open a window to improve the ventilation in the cabin. Simple bedside tests such as a blood glucose level and an ECG will exclude many significant causes. An ECG can uncover dysrhythmias, ischaemia, electrolyte abnormalities and features of anticholinergic poisoning.

Patients with carbon monoxide poisoning can have unfavourable cognitive sequelae, so early diagnosis and management is essential. Hyperbaric oxygen (HBO) is one recommended treatment for acute carbon monoxide poisoning, and indications for treatment include:

- loss of consciousness at any stage;
- age > 50 years;
- carboxyhaemoglobin > 25%;
- metabolic acidosis.

The *New England Journal of Medicine* unequivocally stated in a 2002 article: 'Hyperbaric oxygen treatments within 24 hours after acute carbon monoxide poisoning should be the standard of care' (Piantadosi 2002). However, a 2005 Cochrane review stated that there is no evidence to support use of HBO for treatment of patients with carbon monoxide poisoning (Juurlink et al. 2005). There has been much debate surrounding this topic in recent years. Nevertheless, the precautionary principle is usually applied and if a chamber is readily accessible then the treatment is invariably offered.

Hyperbaric oxygen chambers are available only in some centres, so consultation with the hyperbaric consultant and transport to the centre may be necessary. Patients not fulfilling the treatment criteria may be treated with 100% normobaric oxygen for 72 hours.

Patients with an altered mental state may require advanced airway management (intubation and ventilation) so that the procedure can be carried out safely.

12:45 hours

Frank is reviewed by the hyperbaric oxygen specialist and he is accepted for therapy. He is intubated in the emergency department and is transferred to the hyperbaric chamber to begin his treatment.

Physiology comment

Physiological basis of carbon monoxide toxicity

Carbon monoxide chemically combines with haem-binding sites in the same way as oxygen and therefore reduces the capacity of the blood to carry oxygen. Carbon monoxide has an affinity for haem-binding sites approximately 250 times that of oxygen, forming carboxyhaemoglobin. Carbon monoxide will therefore out-compete oxygen, meaning that, when present, less Hb is able to bind oxygen and therefore deliver oxygen to the tissues. With reference to the definition of Hb saturation, the PaO_2 may well be normal or even elevated (with oxygen treatment), leading to a high level of saturation, but saturation tells us only about the number of available binding sites that are occupied and not about the oxygen content of the blood. Remember also that, when bound, carbon monoxide shifts the dissociation curve to the left, making any oxygen that is present less available to the peripheral tissues.

Carbon monoxide poisoning not only reduces oxygen delivery and availability at the level of the working tissues, but also interferes with cellular processes linked with metabolism, further exacerbating the situation.

Signs and symptoms

The carboxyhaemoglobin level in a healthy non-smoker is usually less than 1.5% unless exposed to environmental carbon monoxide (typically car emissions or cigarette smoke). Heavy smokers can have carboxy-haemoglobin levels as high as 15%. The carboxyhaemoglobin of people suffering from carbon monoxide poisoning is unusually high, typically >20%. It is important to note that in carbon monoxide poisoning the PaO_2 is often normal when breathing air and high when oxygen is administered, but the oxygen content of the blood will be reduced.

A definitive diagnosis of carbon monoxide poisoning comes with the measurement of high levels of carboxyhaemoglobin, with values in poisoning ranging from 20% (mild symptoms) to 60% (coma). As carbon monoxide poisoning reduces oxygen delivery and availability at the level of the working tissues the signs and symptoms of carbon monoxide poisoning are related to tissue hypoxia. The hypoxia may crucially affect the heart (ECG abnormalities leading to cardiac failure and/or myocardial infarction), lungs (hyperventilation and pulmonary oedema), nervous system (peripheral nerve damage and paralysis) and brain (drowsiness, agitation and confusion). As carboxyhaemoglobin is bright red in colour patients may appear to be well perfused and oxygenated with bright red skin, but this isn't always seen, especially if circulatory collapse is coexistent.

Physiological basis of treatment

Treatment for carbon monoxide poisoning is aimed at relieving tissue hypoxia by converting carboxyhaemoglobin to oxyhaemoglobin via administration of oxygen therapy (normobaric or hyperbaric). Oxygen therapy increases the PO_2 in the blood, facilitating the displacement of carbon monoxide with oxygen and to some extent increasing the amount transported as dissolved oxygen. The rate of displacement of carbon monoxide from haemoglobin increases with the PO_2 of the inspired gas and is the basis of hyperbaric therapy. Oxygen therapy is therefore a mainstay of any treatment protocol.

Epilogue

Frank had three oxygen treatments in the hyperbaric chamber in a period of 24 hours and was subsequently extubated and discharged from the intensive care unit. He said he had gone inside into his cabin to work on his motor, but failed to open any windows.

He returned to his previously active life and has suffered no apparent cognitive injury. He still goes out on his boat, but never alone and always with a well-ventilated cabin.

References and further reading

1 Hew, R. Altered conscious state. In Cameron, P. et al. (eds), *Textbook of Adult Emergency Medicine*. 2nd edn. Churchill Livingstone, 2004.
2 Juurlink, D.N., Buckley, N.A., Stanbrook, M.B. et al. Hyperbaric oxygen for carbon monoxide poisoning. The Cochrane Database of Systematic Reviews 2005; Issue 1. Art. No. CD002041.
3 Piantadosi, C.A. Carbon monoxide poisoning. N Engl J Med 2002; 347(14): 1054–5.
4 Weaver, L.K. et al. Hyperbaric oxygen for acute carbon monoxide poisoning. N Engl J Med 2002; 347(14): 1057–67.

Review

Level 1: Content knowledge

1   Dalton's law states that the:
   A   Total pressure of a gas mixture equals the sum of the pressures exerted by each component
   B   Total pressure of a gas mixture equals the pressures exerted by the most abundant component
   C   Volume of a gas mixture equals the sum of the volumes of each component
   D   Total mass of a gas mixture equals the sum of the masses of each component

2   The haemoglobin saturation is:
   A   Amount of oxygen bound to the haem-binding site
   B   Total amount of oxygen carried in the blood
   C   Percentage of oxygen carried in the blood
   D   Percentage of haem-binding sites that have been occupied

3   The sigmoid shape of the oxyhaemoglobin dissociation curve can be explained in part by which of the following?
   A   After the binding of oxygen to haem the affinity of the next binding site for oxygen increases.
   B   After the binding of oxygen to haem the affinity of the next binding site for oxygen decreases.
   C   The limited number of binding sites on the haem.
   D   After the binding of oxygen to haem more binding sites for oxygen become available.

Level 2: Clinical applications

1   Match the following causes of a reduced mental state with the most appropriate clinical findings:
   A   Heroin overdose
   B   Atrial fibrillation with rapid ventricular response
   C   Intracerebral haemorrhage
   D   Diabetic ketoacidosis
   E   Meningococcal sepsis
   F   Carbon monoxide poisoning
      (i)   Significantly dehydrated, rapid breathing, 'acetone' odour on breath
      (ii) Weak pulse, purpuric rash over body
      (iii) Cyanosed, pinpoint pupils

    (iv) Unconscious, few clinical features

    (v) Dilated pupil, high blood pressure, low pulse

    (vi) Irregular weak pulse, low blood pressure

2 Which of the following situations would be the *least* likely to have carbon monoxide poisoning as a cause for a reduced mental state?

  A Unconscious young male rescued from a house fire

  B Semi-conscious male found in a parked motor vehicle

  C Elderly male found unconscious in car at busy intersection

  D Elderly woman found unconscious in house in winter

  E Antarctic explorer found confused in field hut

3 Which of the following findings are indications for treatment with hyperbaric oxygen?

  A Reduced conscious state

  B COHb of 31%

  C Frequent ventricular ectopic beats on ECG

  D Pregnant female with a COHb of 15% and no loss of consciousness

  E All of the above are indications for treatment

Level 3: Topics for further discussion

1 Carbon monoxide poisoning and treatment with hyperbaric oxygen has attracted much attention in the medical literature in recent years. Discuss the advantages and disadvantages of providing such treatment.

2 Discuss the neuropsychological sequelae that may result from carbon monoxide poisoning.

Case 6
Norman barely made it to hospital alive ...

This 72-year-old man presents unexpectedly to the hospital with difficulties breathing and then rapidly deteriorates. Your life-saving skills, combined with a working knowledge of cardiovascular physiology, allow you to institute life-saving definitive therapy and save his life.

Timeline summary

19:00	Onset of chest pain and breathlessness at home; decides to drive to hospital.
19:18	Arrives at hospital; rushed into monitored bed; basic support commenced.
19:21	Clinical diagnosis considered; specific therapy commenced.
19:30	12-lead electrocardiogram (ECG) and chest X-ray (CXR) obtained.
19:35	Deterioration and intubation.
19:50	Arterial line inserted and first arterial blood gas (ABG) obtained.
19:55	Second CXR taken to check endotracheal tube position.
20:05	Cardiologist attends and performs bedside echocardiography.
20:20	Second ABG.
20:45	Transfer to Intensive Care Unit (ICU).

Learning objectives

Physiological

- Describe the two main categories of pulmonary oedema.
- Outline the determinants of rate of fluid accumulation in lung.
- Describe how the Starling's forces might alter to favour pulmonary oedema.

- Understand why the key determinant of cardiogenic pulmonary oedema is an increase in left aortic pressure.
- Explain how pulmonary oedema may alter lung mechanics and gas exchange.
- Understand the physiological basis of treatment for pulmonary oedema.

Clinical

- Understand the principles of diagnosis and management of the patient with severe breathlessness.
- Describe the therapies available to use in the Emergency Department for the patient with acutely decompensated congestive cardiac failure (CCF).
- Describe the causes and precipitants of acute pulmonary oedema.

Context

Norman barely made it to hospital alive. Normally quite well, he complained of chest heaviness at around 7:00 p.m. He felt breathless and sweaty, and decided to drive himself to the hospital 15 minutes away from home.

19:18 hours

The triage nurse at the front desk takes one look at him and makes him a 'category 2' patient.

'Patients this sick usually arrive by ambulance', he thinks to himself.

Norman is rapidly ushered into a bed in the Emergency Department and nursing staff apply oxygen and monitoring. Looking particularly grey and unwell, he is reassigned 'category 1', and the resuscitation staff are called to attend.

Norman looks really sick. He can barely say two words, and he is sweating so profusely that monitoring dots will not stick to him. The consultant applies his stethoscope to his chest: coarse crackles can be heard throughout his left and right lung fields. As the nursing staff prepare for intravenous cannulation and an ECG, a brief history is taken in response to directed questions:

' … heaviness across my chest … can't breathe … no allergies … Diabex, Losec …'

19:21 hours

The monitors provide much needed information and, while intravenous cannulation is occurring, radiography is contacted for an urgent mobile CXR. The following information becomes available:

- PR: 130 bpm
- BP: 260/140 mmHg
- RR: 40 breaths/min
- SpO_2:   unable to be determined (presumably due to poor peripheral perfusion)

Clinical question 1

The above has taken place in a matter of just 5 minutes.

(a) What are you thinking?

(b) What is your differential diagnosis?

Clinical comment

As the mobile CXR was being taken the diagnosis was apparent to all: acute pulmonary oedema, possibly produced by acute myocardial ischaemia or hypertension.

Norman looks seriously ill. The consultant is concerned and rapidly initiates emergency treatment.

'Let's start a glyceryl trinitrate infusion, and give him an aspirin. And could we get the CPAP machine and get it started, but let's also be prepared to intubate him if there's no immediate response.'

Clinical comment

This patient clinically has pulmonary oedema, and if treatment can be started rapidly with intravenous glyceryl trinitrate and continuous positive airway pressure (CPAP) he may be able to survive this acute phase of the illness. Patients often rapidly respond to physiological manipulation of the preload and afterload, but they must be observed closely and new plans must be quickly developed and implemented in response to changes in the patient's condition if necessary.

19:30 hours

A 12-lead ECG is produced (see Fig. 6.1).

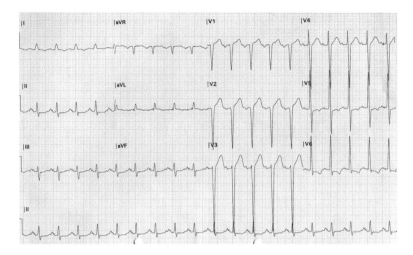

Figure 6.1 ECG

The radiographer returns with the chest X-ray (see Fig. 6.2).

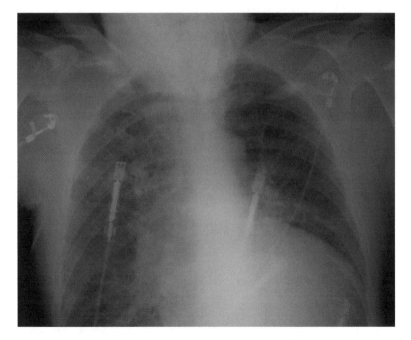

Figure 6.2 First chest X-ray

Clinical question 2

(a) Interpret the CXR.
(b) Interpret the ECG.

Clinical comment

The ECG shows a sinus tachycardia with diagnostic features of left ventricular hypertrophy, as evidenced by deep S waves in V_{1-4} and tall R waves in V_{5-6}. The T-wave inversion in the lateral leads (I, aVL, V_{5-6}) may also represent left ventricular hypertrophy, but could represent acute myocardial ischaemia.

The CXR has many of the features that would be expected given the clinical presentation: the increased whiteness in the lung fields represents interstitial oedema, and there is significant cardiomegaly.

Physiology comment

Pulmonary oedema is the abnormal accumulation of fluid in the interstitial spaces surrounding alveoli, with possible fluid exudation into alveolar air space. Pulmonary oedema can be usefully categorised into two main categories based upon the physiological cause:

• high pressure, hydrostatic and cardiogenic refer to an elevated pulmonary capillary hydrostatic cause; and
• low pressure, high permeability and non-cardiogenic refer to conditions where permeability is elevated.

19:35 hours

Norman is clearly tiring, and his breathing is becoming shallower. He appeared drowsier than before.

'He's not responding,' says the nurse.

'I agree,' says the consultant, 'We're going to have to intubate him. It's a shame … I thought the therapy was going to work.'

Norman is transferred to the resuscitation room where the medical and nursing team prepare to escalate treatment. Preparations for intubation are commenced, drugs are drawn up and roles allocated.

The intubating doctor inserts a size 8 endotracheal tube, with some difficulty:

'There's a lot of frothy fluid coming up, I can hardly see a thing', he comments.

Nevertheless, the tube is successfully passed between the cords and a reassuring pattern appears on the monitor (see Fig. 6.3).

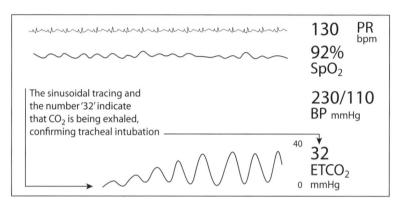

Figure 6.3 Capnography tracing end-tidal PCO_2

Clinical question 3

How can you be sure the trachea has been intubated in this situation?

 ### Clinical comment

Airway management is an essential skill for emergency physicians, and endotracheal intubation is a procedure that, while being potentially life-saving, can carry a high mortality if carried out incorrectly. Oesophageal intubation is a risk that must be recognised early if complications and possible death are to be avoided. The intubating doctor can use a number of techniques to confirm that the trachea has been intubated, and these include direct visualisation, auscultation of breath sounds, and misting of the endotracheal tube during ventilation. However, these techniques have limitations, and the use of capnography (end-tidal PCO_2) and oesophageal detector devices are more reliable and should be used routinely.

The situation has stabilised somewhat, but Norman is still critically ill.

'We need to hyperventilate him as I imagine he's really acidotic and we need to maintain the respiratory compensation.'

The airway nurse asks, 'What settings would you like on the ventilator?'

The consultant replies, 'I'd like to start on a respiratory rate of 18 with 8 of PEEP. Let's see how the blood pressure tolerates that and we'll reassess.' (See Fig. 6.4.)

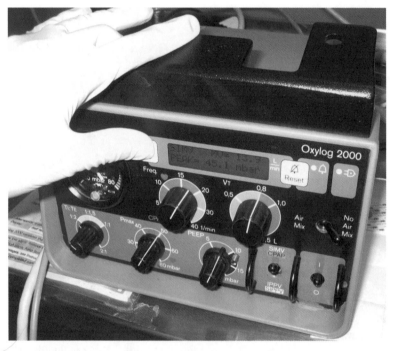

Figure 6.4 Ventilator settings

19:50 hours

An arterial line is placed so that arterial blood can be sampled frequently and blood pressure can be closely monitored. Together with the patient's clinical state, the monitoring indicates an improvement in the parameters (see Fig. 6.5).

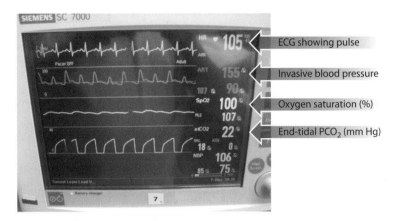

Figure 6.5 Monitor readings

The first ABG taken after intubation showed the results in Table 6.1.

Table 6.1 Arterial blood gas results

FIO_2	1.0
Blood gas values:	
pH	7.276
$PaCO_2$	45.6 mmHg
PaO_2	444 mmHg
Base excess	−6.0 mmol/L
HCO_3^-	20.6 mmol/L
Oximetry values:	
Hb	157 g/L
SaO_2	99.3%
Electrolyte values:	
K^+	3.4 mmol/L
Na^+	136 mmol/L
Metabolite values:	
Glu	13.7 mmol/L
Lac	3.4 mmol/L

Clinical question 4

(a) Interpret the ABG results and comment.

(b) Will you adjust the ventilation settings?

(c) How?

Clinical comment

The patient was initially suffering cardiogenic shock; he presumably had a metabolic acidosis and, due to his laboured breathing, a degree of acute respiratory acidosis. Now that he has been intubated and ventilated it is essential to take his compensation requirements into account. His $PaCO_2$ is still elevated at 46 mmHg—to compensate for the underlying metabolic acidosis it is necessary to hyperventilate him and monitor his acid–base status closely. Increasing the respiratory rate or the tidal volume increases alveolar ventilation. The tidal volume will need to be adjusted carefully based upon the measured airway pressures: high pressures increase the risk of causing barotrauma, and a pneumothorax at this stage would serve only to further complicate an already critical situation.

19:55 hours

Once the patient is intubated, a better quality CXR is obtained (see Fig. 6.6).

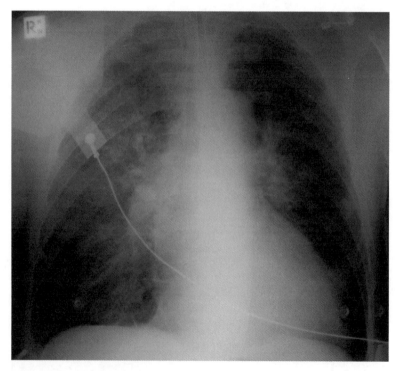

Figure 6.6 Second chest X-ray

20:05 hours

The emergency consultant has been in early contact with the on-call cardiologist. The ECG has not shown any indications for reperfusion therapy, and the cardiologist attends the department to perform bedside echocardiography on the patient.

The cardiologist looks intently at the monitor and then at the patient.

'I agree, there's nothing on the ECG to suggest we should take him to the lab for an urgent angioplasty, but the echocardiogram shows a thickened left ventricle. I think he's had poorly managed hypertension and tonight he had an acute hypertensive crisis and he decompensated.'

At this stage things have stabilised: his blood pressure has settled, his chest is sounding much clearer, his heart rate is settling. All he has to do now is to survive this acute episode, and he is showing every indication that he will. A bed is arranged in the ICU, and preparations are made to transfer him there (see Fig. 6.7).

Infusions and monitoring, ready for transport

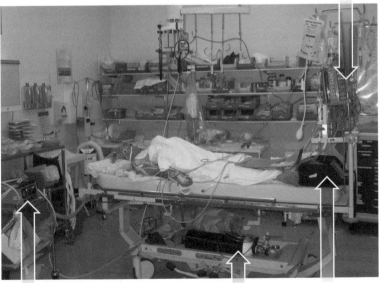

Ventilator

Portable oxygen cylinder

Defibrillator

Figure 6.7 The patient ready for transfer to ICU

20:20 hours

Prior to transfer to the ICU a repeat ABG is done to check the adequacy of the new ventilation settings (see Table 6.2).

Table 6.2 Second arterial blood gas results

FIO_2	1.0
Blood gas values:	
pH	7.398
$PaCO_2$	36.2 mmHg
PaO_2	411 mmHg
Base excess	−1.9 mmol/L
HCO_3^-	21.8 mmol/L
Oximetry values:	
Hb	151 g/L
SaO_2	99.6%
Electrolyte values:	
K^+	3.0 mmol/L
Na^+	136 mmol/L
Ca^{2+}	1.04 mmol/L
Metabolite values:	
Glu	11.2 mmol/L
Lac	1.6 mmol/L

20:45 hours

The patient is transferred to ICU; his condition has stabilised.

Epilogue

Norman spent 2 days in the ICU before he was extubated and transferred to a general medical ward. His blood tests confirmed that he had not had a myocardial infarction, and it was deduced that his acute illness had been precipitated by an acute hypertensive crisis on a background of years of untreated hypertension. He was commenced on appropriate antihypertensive and heart failure therapy (an ACE inhibitor and a β-blocker) and discharged after 6 days in hospital.

Clinical comment

This patient was seriously ill and was lucky to make it to hospital alive. Ideally he would have called an ambulance to attend to him. Ambulance personnel are trained to administer life-saving pre-hospital therapy and can expedite transfer and treatment. The main clinical lesson here is that pre-emptive therapy is essential. The patient was about to have a cardiorespiratory arrest, and early intervention and aggressive therapy prevented this. It is essential to consider the following issues.

Norman was in acute pulmonary oedema and urgent manipulation of the pathophysiological processes at work is essential; hence, the use of venodilators and CPAP has become standard therapy. Venodilators such as intravenous glyceryl trinitrate act to predominantly reduce the preload but also have an effect on the afterload, and CPAP improves left ventricular function and oxygenation. The sum total is to increase cardiac output and reduce the work of breathing. It may be necessary to add specific vasodilators such as hydralazine to reduce the afterload if an adequate response does not occur. A diuretic such as frusemide may have a role in ongoing management if fluid overload is thought to have contributed to the condition.

In this situation the work of breathing became too much, and the patient was becoming obtunded. He needed to be intubated so that he could receive adequate oxygenation and ventilation. Attending to the urgent needs of airway and breathing should not be delayed if initial therapies are clearly not working.

The precipitants of such an acute episode must be identified—ischaemia, hypertension and infection are common precipitants of acute pulmonary oedema in this setting. There were no indications for reperfusion therapy in this instance, but a non-STEMI (ST elevation myocardial infarction) could not be ruled out. Hence, aspirin was administered and an unfractionated heparin infusion was commenced. Further investigations such as angiography can be carried out once the patient has stabilised.

Physiology comment

Determinants of rate of fluid accumulation in lung

Net fluid movement out of the pulmonary capillaries is equal to the filtration coefficient (Kf) × net filtration pressure (NFP). The water permeability and surface area of the capillaries determines Kf, and NFP is determined by the balance of the Starling forces acting across the capillary wall. The following factors therefore determine the rate of fluid accumulation in the lung:

- rate of filtration:
  - capillary forces: hydrostatic and osmotic;
  - permeability;
  - surface area;
- rate of reabsorption:
  - pulmonary lymphatics.

How Starling's forces might alter to favour pulmonary oedema

Pulmonary oedema is favoured if there is an increase in pulmonary capillary pressure, decrease in interstitial pressure, decrease in plasma oncotic pressure or increase in interstitial oncotic pressure. Alterations in Kf may also favour the accumulation of fluid in the lung. An increase in permeability of the capillary endothelium and/or an increase in pulmonary surface area (as seen with increases in cardiac output and pulmonary capillary recruitment) will favour pulmonary oedema.

The key determinant of cardiogenic pulmonary oedema is an increase in left atrial pressure

The patient in this case is experiencing pulmonary oedema that has a primarily cardiogenic cause. Increases in pulmonary capillary pressure (PCP) will favour pulmonary oedema. Increase in PCP can be due to increased left atrial (LA) pressure or increased pulmonary artery pressure. As pulmonary capillary pressure is closer to LA pressure than pulmonary artery pressure, due to the distribution of resistance in the pulmonary capillary bed, the key determinant of cardiogenic pulmonary oedema is an increase in LA pressure. Systolic (contraction) failure and/or diastolic (compliance) failure are common causes of elevated LA pressure. Either systolic or diastolic failure, or a combination of both, may have led to the increased PCP in this case.

Lung mechanics

Pulmonary interstitial pressure is negative under normal conditions due to alveolar surface tension. Alveolar surface tension causes the alveoli to collapse in on themselves; however, due to the fact that they are tethered together, the pressure in the spaces between the alveoli (interstitial spaces, Pint) is relatively negative. The Pint therefore favours accumulation of fluid in the interstitium; if effectiveness of surfactant is reduced, accumulation of fluid may be further favoured. Surfactant can be lost if pulmonary oedema becomes severe due to dilution and physical rupture of the alveoli.

The dilution of surfactant reduces the compliance of the alveoli. The lungs are normally very compliant (compliance = $\Delta V/\Delta P$), which enables ventilation to occur with relatively little energy expenditure.

If pulmonary oedema occurs then lung compliance is reduced ('stiff lungs') and the work of breathing increases (work = $\Delta V \times \Delta P$). A decrease in lung compliance, decreased lung volume (caused by a collapse of alveoli and alveolar filling) and remaining alveoli having to distend further to accommodate tidal volume all lead to an increased work of breathing. Clinically this increased work of breathing manifests with the patient taking shallow tidal volumes with a fast respiratory rate.

Gas exchange

There are several mechanisms by which pulmonary oedema may lead to a reduction in gas exchange. Reduced lung volume caused by collapsed or fluid filled alveoli lead to unventilated, but perfused, regions of the lung (in effect a right-to-left shunt is occurring). Decreased ventilation in well-perfused areas also leads to V/Q mismatching, which reduces gas exchange. Accumulation of fluid in the interstitial space increases the thickness of the alveolar capillary membrane, further reducing the effectiveness of gas exchange. All these factors coupled with reduced total ventilation mean that hypoxaemia is a major concern in pulmonary oedema.

Understand the physiological basis of treatment

The normo- or hypertensive patient suffering from pulmonary oedema needs to sit upright (decreasing venous return), be given oxygen and nitrates (venodilation) and also given non-invasive ventilatory support. This therapy is aimed at reducing PCP (the cause of the pulmonary oedema) while supplying the patient with oxygen and ventilatory support.

References and further reading

1   Crane, S.D., Elliott, M.W., Gilligan, P., Richards, K. and Gray, A.J. Randomised controlled comparison of continuous positive airways pressure, bilevel non-invasive ventilation, and standard treatment in emergency department patients with acute cardiogenic pulmonary oedema. Emerg Med J 2004; 21: 155–61.

2   Fonarow, G.C., Corday, E. and the ADHERE Scientific Advisory Committee. Overview of acutely decompensated congestive heart failure (ADHF): A report from the ADHERE registry. Heart Fail Rev 2005 Jan; 9(3): 179–85.

3   Graham, C.A. Pharmacological therapy of acute cardiogenic pulmonary oedema in the emergency department. Emergency Medicine Australasia 2004; 16: 47–54.

4   Peacock, W.F. Acute emergency department management of heart failure. Heart Fail Rev 2003 Oct; 8(4): 335–8.

5   Wakai, A., McMahon, G. Nitrates for acute heart failure. (Protocol.) The Cochrane Database of Systematic Reviews 2005; Issue 1. Art. No. CD005151.

Review

Level 1: Content knowledge

1 Cardiogenic pulmonary oedema is best defined as:
   A Development of pulmonary oedema as a consequence of increased capillary hydrostatic pressure, secondary to elevated left atrial pressure
   B Development of pulmonary oedema as a consequence of increased interstitial hydrostatic pressure, secondary to elevated left atrial pressure
   C Development of pulmonary oedema as a consequence of increased capillary permeability, secondary to acute inflammation
   D Development of pulmonary oedema as a consequence of decreased capillary oncotic pressure, secondary to liver failure

2 In pulmonary oedema, the lungs become:
   A Less compliant and the functional residual capacity increases
   B Less compliant and the functional residual capacity decreases
   C More compliant and the functional residual capacity increases
   D More compliant and the functional residual capacity decreases

3 High permeability oedema:
   A Is characterised by an increase in the reflection coefficient
   B Can be caused by multiple trauma remote from the lungs
   C Leads to a dilution of surfactant and an increase in compliance
   D Can be caused by a blockage of the lymphatic system

Level 2: Clinical applications

1 Which of the following treatments are *not* currently recommended for the emergency management of acute pulmonary oedema?
   A CPAP
   B Glyceryl trinitrate infusion
   C Frusemide
   D BiPAP
   E Oxygen

2 Which of the following agents would be of most benefit in a patient with acute pulmonary oedema and a blood pressure of 260/140 mmHg resistant to a glyceryl trinitrate infusion?
   A Morphine
   B Frusemide
   C Hydralazine
   D Metoprolol
   E Intravenous verapamil

3 Which of the following clinical signs are *not* suggestive of acute pulmonary oedema as a cause of a patient's breathlessness?

A Bilateral wheezes and crackles on auscultation
B Raised respiratory rate with signs of respiratory distress
C Fourth heart sound
D Diaphoretic patient
E Clear chest on auscultation

Level 3: Topics for further discussion

1 Morphine and frusemide are still recommended as having roles in the acute management of pulmonary oedema. Review the evidence and discuss their roles.

2 Discuss the possible precipitants of acute pulmonary oedema and how you would identify and manage them in the Emergency Department.

Case 7
An elderly man collapses
at home …

This 75-year-old patient collapses and is poorly perfused. The cause is not immediately apparent, as there are a number of possible physiological explanations for his condition. The patient's condition rapidly deteriorates and resuscitation begins.

Timeline summary

18:52	Collapse at home; wife rings ambulance.
19:20	Arrives at the Emergency Department.
19:23–19:35	Intubation, resuscitation, emergency ultrasonography; chest X-ray (CXR).
19:35	Therapy directed towards correcting cardiogenic shock.
19:41	12-lead electrocardiogram (ECG) obtained; deterioration into ventricular fibrillation and cardiac arrest; onset of advanced cardiac life support (ACLS).
19:50	Deteriorates into asystole.
19:57	Resuscitation withdrawn and patient declared deceased.

Learning objectives

Physiological

- Understand how the development of oedema is linked with cardiac failure.
- Understand the concept of 'anion gap' and state how it would be altered in this case.
- State Starling's law, the principles of preload and afterload, and their effects on cardiac output, and how they relate to this case.

Clinical

- Describe the emergency management of the shocked patient, regardless of the cause.
- Understand the factors that contribute to cardiogenic shock.
- Know the basic life support (BLS) and ACLS protocols in use in your region.
- Be able to utilise electrocardiography to diagnose ischaemic heart disease and rhythm disturbances.

Context

The triage nurse comes into the staff station with news that an ambulance is 5 minutes away with a 75-year-old Mr White, who collapsed at home. He is now conscious but hypotensive; he's sweaty and looks unwell. He has a distended abdomen. Oxygen is being administered by facemask and they are proceeding rapidly to the Emergency Department. No other information is available.

Clinical question 1

(a) What will you do to prepare for his arrival?

(b) Make a list of equipment that you may need to use in this situation.

(c) Which staff will you notify in advance to assist with his resuscitation?

(d) Discuss your differential diagnoses based on the information you have at this stage.

You proceed to the resuscitation room and begin to prepare for Mr White's arrival—intravenous cannulae and fluids are prepared, the airway equipment is checked, and the radiology staff is pre-warned.

19:20 hours

The patient arrives on a stretcher and looks unwell; he is conscious, but is sweating profusely. He is struggling to breathe, and he has an obviously distended abdomen. He can hardly speak, so little history is available from him directly. Oxygen therapy is continued at 15 L/min via a non-rebreathing mask.

The vital signs and initial examination become readily apparent during the primary survey:

- He looks pale and sweaty.
- PR: 95 bpm
- RR: 30 breaths/min and shallow
- BP: 110/95 mmHg
- GCS: 13 (E4, V4, M5)
- The chest has widespread coarse crackles throughout both lung fields.

The consultant takes handover from the paramedic:

'His wife said he'd been getting increasingly unwell over the last 36 hours—more breathless, his abdomen becoming more distended. It got worse and he collapsed around 30 minutes ago, complaining of abdominal pain and left shoulder pain, and that's when she called us. He has a history of hypertension and heart disease, having had bypass surgery 6 years ago'.

Further examination reveals the following:

- His abdomen is markedly distended.
- Femoral pulses are weak and his popliteal pulses are barely palpable, and the pulses in his feet are unable to be palpated.
- There is bilateral pitting oedema to above his knees.

Clinical question 2

Having assessed the patient, what would be your differential diagnosis now?

19:23–19:35 hours

Meanwhile, Mr White's breathing is becoming increasingly difficult and laboured. Given his shocked state a decision is made to secure his airway and intubate him. The airway doctor pre-oxygenates the patient with 100% oxygen and a resident doctor inserts a wide-bore intravenous cannula into his left ante-cubital fossa, and collects blood simultaneously.

A rapid sequence induction occurs, and the patient is intubated with a size 9 endotracheal tube. The patient is ventilated by hand on 100% oxygen, and a resident doctor takes an arterial blood sample for analysis.

The consultant has decided that a ruptured abdominal aortic aneurysm is a possible diagnosis, and performs a bedside emergency ultrasound scan on the patient. However, because of the patient's physique, very little can be seen on the ultrasound.

A CXR is rapidly obtained post-intubation (see Fig. 7.1).

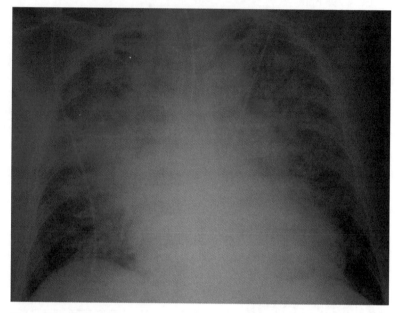

Figure 7.1 Chest X-ray

Clinical question 3

(a) Comment on the CXR. List the main features.
(b) Does this CXR provide you with any information that will alter your management?

Clinical comment

The patient is seriously unwell; he is shocked and he has a distended abdomen. Given his history of abdominal pain and collapse it is important to think of a ruptured abdominal aortic aneurysm. He also has clinical signs of pulmonary oedema. Worsening biventricular failure over the preceding days could explain his peripheral oedema and distended abdomen. The CXR shows gross cardiomegaly and pulmonary oedema; and with his history of ischaemic heart disease the shock is most likely cardiogenic in origin. At this stage the acute precipitant of his current state remains unknown.

Physiology comment

Remember from Case 1 that shock can be defined as inadequate tissue perfusion as a result of depressed cardiac output. Shock can be usefully categorised based upon the cause of the drop in cardiac output:

- hypovolemic (low circulating volume);
- cardiogenic (decreased cardiac performance);
- distributive (normal blood volume but vasodilation);
- obstructive (impediment to blood flow).

Which physiological classification of shock do you think the patient falls into? If shock progresses into a decompensated phase no matter what the initial cause of shock it will almost always progress to having a cardiogenic component. Why do you think this is the case?

Fluid movement across the capillary (systemic or pulmonary) endothelium is governed by the balance of Starling's forces (hydrostatic and oncotic: osmotic force due to the plasma proteins in the blood). Elevated venous pressure due to an inability of the heart to pump blood into the high-pressure side of the circulation will result in congestion and elevated venous pressures. The resultant imbalance of Starling's forces leads to an increased filtration out of the capillaries, leading to the collection of fluid in the interstitial space (oedema). Initial left ventricular failure will result in raised pulmonary pressure and therefore pulmonary oedema, whereas initial right heart failure will lead to a raised central venous pressure and peripheral oedema. Left- or right-sided heart failure, if left untreated, will eventually lead to failure of the other side once compensatory mechanisms are overwhelmed. What is important is that the order of occurrence and progression of any oedema can give clues to the side of heart that has failed initially.

The ABG is available (see Table 7.1).

Table 7.1 Arterial blood gas results

FIO_2	1.0
Blood gas values:	
pH	7.062
$PaCO_2$	30.1 mmHg
PaO_2	195 mmHg
BE	−20.9 mmol/L
HCO_3^-	9.3 mmol/L
Oximetry values:	
Hb	103 g/L
SaO_2	98.3%
Electrolyte values:	
K^+	5.0 mmol/L
Na^+	137 mmol/L
Ca^+	1.39 mmol/L
Ca^{2+} (7.4)	1.14 mmol/L
Metabolite values:	
Glu	10.1 mmol/L
Lac	9.4 mmol/L

Clinical question 4

(a) Interpret the arterial blood gas data and calculate his $P(A-a)O_2$ gradient.

(b) Will you adjust the ventilator settings based on this result?

 Physiology comment

There are two basic types of metabolic acidosis and they can be readily distinguished by evaluating the anion gap. One type of metabolic acidosis leads to an unchanged anion gap and the other leads to an increased anion gap.

The sum of the negative charges in a solution always balances the sum of the positive charges. However, not every ionic constituent of the plasma is normally reported by the laboratory. Often only sodium, chloride and bicarbonate are given.

Therefore the balance of positive and negative charges in solution is given by:

$$[Na^+] + [other\ cations] = [HCO_3^-] + [Cl^-] + [other\ anions]$$

The difference between the unreported cations and anions is equal to ([sodium] – ([bicarbonate] + [chloride]) and is termed the 'anion gap'. The anion gap is normally 8–16 mEq/L and is useful in the differential diagnosis of acid–base disorders.

In the case of increased anaerobic metabolism due to inadequate oxygenation of the blood or decreased tissue perfusion, lactic acid accumulates in the plasma. The increasing levels of lactate lead to a fall in bicarbonate; this buffering goes some way to blunt the drop in pH. As the bicarbonate levels have fallen and the chloride levels have remained unchanged the anion gap increases. An increasing anion gap therefore indicates the presence of a new acid anion in the plasma. Examples of such acid anions are lactate (in lactic acidosis), acetoacetate, beta-OH butyrate (diabetic acidosis, starvation ketosis) or salicylate (salicylate poisoning).

Loss of bicarbonate from the gastrointestinal tract can also lead to the development of a metabolic acidosis. In this case, however, the anion gap remains unchanged as the loss of bicarbonate is balanced by an increase in chloride (hyperchloraemia). The sodium bicarbonate lost in diarrhoea fluid is replaced by sodium chloride through renal reabsorption and/or infusion.

19:35 hours

Mr White's blood pressure remains low, his pulse rate is still 90 bpm, and he is being hyperventilated.

Mr White remains seriously ill; it appears that he is in cardiogenic shock, a condition that carries a high mortality. A 12-lead ECG is obtained in an attempt to identify a precipitant. Fluid resuscitation continues in an attempt to improve perfusion. However, the consultant recognises that with a failing heart the patient will require inotropic support combined with treatment of the cause.

'We need to set up for a central line and prepare a noradrenaline infusion. We'll also need to insert an arterial line. But let's try to improve his perfusion first.'

19:41 hours

The ECG is handed to the consultant (see Fig. 7.2).

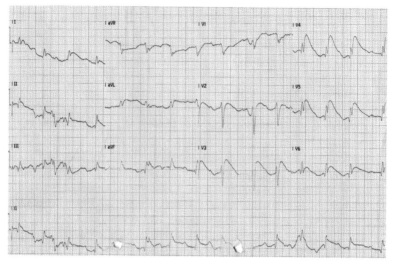

Figure 7.2 12-lead ECG

Clinical question 5

(a) Despite the interference, can this ECG be interpreted?
(b) Does it provide you with a reason for the patient's condition?
(c) What treatment should be considered?

However, before any intervention can be started, the patient takes a turn for the worse. The heart monitor, which up until now has been beeping regularly, suddenly changes and reveals the rhythm shown in Figure 7.3.

There is no palpable pulse at this time—the rhythm is ventricular fibrillation and the patient is in cardiac arrest.

'Commence chest compressions', calls the consultant, 'and defibrillate with 150 joules from the biphasic defibrillator.'

One litre of 0.9% normal saline is rapidly infused into the patient through the intravenous cannula; a medical student is performing external cardiac massage as per BLS protocols. The patient is defibrillated a further four times, but remains in ventricular fibrillation. The rhythm strip is difficult to assess while CPR is taking place; after the fifth shock from the defibrillator the team leader asks for chest compressions to pause briefly so the rhythm can be properly assessed.

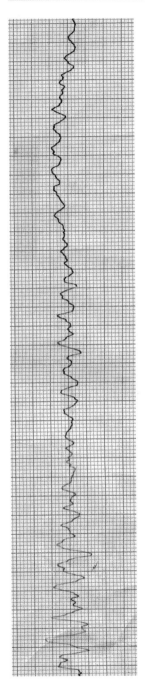

Figure 7.3 ECG rhythm strip demonstrating ventricular fibrillation

19:50 hours

The patient is in asystole.

'This is looking grim', says the consultant. 'But let's continue CPR—keep giving 1 mg of adrenaline every 3 minutes, and could we please give 1 mg of atropine immediately.'

Clinical question 6

What is the prognosis of patients once this condition occurs?

19:57 hours

Mr White remains in asystole despite recommended interventions, and further resuscitation attempts are deemed to be futile. The patient is declared deceased.

Clinical comment

This patient presented acutely unwell; however, despite him not having an immediate apparent diagnosis urgent interventions were required to keep him alive. The early intubation was important: he was working hard at breathing and he was clearly underperfused. A paradox of treatment was apparent: he was obviously fluid overloaded, but shocked: how can we acutely manage him? It may seem counter-intuitive to treat him with fluid boluses, but do remember that it takes time to insert a central line and commence inotropes. Fluid remains the first step in the management of shock, whatever the cause—it can be given quickly and relatively safely. The fact is that this patient deteriorated so rapidly that inotropes were unable to be started. He received adrenaline and atropine in the context of receiving ACLS.

The distended abdomen, combined with a story of abdominal pain and collapse led to the initial diagnosis of ruptured aortic aneurysm being considered, producing hypovolaemic shock. The diagnosis of cardiogenic shock was considered only after the CXR was viewed: however, this coincided with both the diagnosis of an anterior myocardial infarction and his rapid deterioration into ventricular fibrillation.

Most causes of pulmonary oedema and exacerbation of cardiac failure have a definable cause. In addition to treating the condition it is essential to identify and treat any such precipitants. In this circumstance the ECG was diagnostic of an acute myocardial infarction. Unfortunately in practice the ECG is never as neat and tidy as those usually published in textbooks: in an emergency situation the clinician often has to elicit the information from substandard data. Nevertheless, marked S-T elevation diagnostic of an acute myocardial infarction can be seen in the anterior leads of the ECG (mainly V3–V6). However, the patient was never stable enough for reperfusion therapy to be administered, either by thrombolysis or percutaneous coronary intervention (PCI). Published evidence supports the use of PCI in patients with cardiogenic shock, Aggressive therapy with inotropes and intra-aortic balloon pumping is recommended to support cardiac output and can reduce mortality.

Other precipitants of acute cardiac failure include:

- systemic hypertension;
- dysrhythmia;
- systemic infection;
- anaemia;
- acute myocarditis;
- acute valvular dysfunction;
- pulmonary embolus;
- pharmacologic complications (such as alteration of drug therapy).

It seems unlikely that Mr White would have survived whatever the situation. Acute myocardial infarction complicated by cardiogenic shock carries a high mortality in excess of 50%. He had been becoming progressively more unwell over a 36-hour period. It would have been ideal to have seen him in the Emergency Department earlier in the course of his illness. When he finally arrested it was on the background of progressively worsening cardiac failure leading to cardiogenic shock. His final rhythm of asystole represents the terminal progression of his condition: the heart muscle is so badly damaged that the cells are no longer functioning and are unable to respond to any further treatment. Asystole is the natural end-point of no cardiac perfusion, and represents cellular death.

Clinical summary

Presentation

Seventy-five year-old Mr White, with congestive cardiac failure (CCF), presents to the Emergency Department after a collapse.

Tests and results

- ABG showing lactic acidosis.
- CXR showing enlarged heart and pulmonary oedema.
- ECG demonstrating S-T elevation.

Diagnosis

The diagnosis is congestive heart failure, with an acute myocardial infarction (MI) precipitating cardiogenic shock. Clinical signs for diagnosis of CCF include coarse crackles in lungs, distended abdomen (due to ascites as a result of reduced venous return), pitting oedema, reduced or absent leg pulses.

Clinical picture

There was congestive heart failure, leading to fluid overload and resulting in complete cardiac failure and subsequent death. A previous history of cardiac insults combined with hypoxia, fluid retention and oedema to overwhelm the heart's ability to maintain cardiac output, leading to further reductions in cardiac function, worsening hypoxia, fluid retention, and subsequent pulmonary and peripheral oedema. These factors can be seen to combine to create a negative feedback loop that will continue until the heart can no longer cope with the restrictions imposed on its limited abilities. Unless this negative cycle of events is broken, the only result of this is failure of the heart to function and death.

Physiology summary

Determinants of cardiac performance

There are four factors that affect stroke volume:

- contractility;
- venous filling pressure;

- aortic pressure;
- diastolic compliance.

Contractility

When heart muscle is depolarised, insufficient calcium is released to occupy all the troponin C calcium-binding sites. As a result, the force of contraction is less than the theoretical maximum. The calcium concentration and hence contractility can be modulated by stimulation of sympathetic adrenergic β-receptors. If the amount of available calcium is increased, then the force of contraction for any given muscle length (overlap) is increased. This leads to an upwards shift of the systolic pressure curve and a greater force of contraction.

In Mr White's case, however, contractility is depressed rather than increased due to cardiac damage or maladaption. This leads to a reduced force of contraction for any given level of fibre overlap. The primary consequences of this reduction in contractility are a reduced stroke volume, inadequate cardiac output and increased venous pressure. This reduction in contractility can be addressed temporarily by the use of an appropriate cardiac stimulant (inotropic agent). An increased venous pressure is the cardinal sign of heart failure and the pressure rise can be so high that fluid is extruded from the capillaries into the tissues. The resulting peripheral and/or pulmonary oedema can often pose a greater problem than the heart failure itself.

Venous filling pressure

An elevated venous filling pressure can have a deleterious effect upon cardiac performance. The end-diastolic volume is determined by the venous filling pressure. As the ventricles are usually very compliant in health, small changes in filling pressure bring about large changes in diastolic filling volume. Due to this relationship venous filling pressure is a primary determinant of stroke volume and therefore cardiac output. Factors that increase filling pressure usually tend to increase cardiac output and those that decrease venous pressure decrease cardiac output. In Mr White's case the failing heart is unable to increase its stroke volume in response to the elevated filling pressure, contributing to a further rise in right heart and venous pressures and a fall in cardiac output. This inability of the heart to respond to an increased preload is related to dilation of the chamber diameter. Dilation is caused by a slippage of the contractile elements in response to sustained high filling pressures, and means that systolic pressure and stroke volume actually fall with an increasing venous filling pressure.

Aortic pressure

An increase in the aortic pressure will lead to a larger end systolic volume, further leading to a decrease in stroke volume. Thus a rise in aortic pressure tends to decrease stroke volume whereas a falling aortic pressure tends to increase it.

Diastolic compliance

Diastolic compliance cannot be altered during health because in the normal heart the stiffness of the myocytes is determined wholly by the structures that make up their parallel elastic elements. However, diastolic compliance can be altered by disease. When the heart hypertrophies (due to chronic volume or pressure overload), the walls of the ventricle thicken, reducing compliance and thereby reducing diastolic filling.

Key point

As venous pressure is such an important determinant of cardiac performance, a catheter is almost always placed in the critically ill patient (if time allows) to monitor venous pressure and guide patient management. If cardiac output and venous pressure fall, the problem must be one of a depressed circulating volume and appropriate fluids are administered to raise the blood volume. If, however, venous pressure rises as cardiac output falls, then the problem is cardiac in nature and the use of a cardiac stimulant would be more effective. It is obvious in Mr White's case that the initial problem was primarily pump (heart) versus volume related. The pulmonary and venous pressures progressively increased (indicated by the worsening pulmonary and peripheral oedema) as the cardiac output (indicated by the mean arterial pressure) progressively fell.

References and further reading

1 Hochman, J.S., Sleeper, L.A., Webb, J.G. et al. Early revascularization in acute myocardial infarction complicated by cardiogenic shock. N Engl J Med 1999 Aug 26; 341(9): 625–34.
2 The International Liaison Committee on Resuscitation (ILCOR) publishes up-to-date guidelines and information regarding resuscitation. http://www.c2005.org
3 Randomized trial of intravenous streptokinase, oral aspirin, both, or neither among 17,187 cases of suspected acute myocardial infarction: ISIS-2. ISIS-2 (Second International Study of Infarct Survival) Collaborative Group. J Am Coll Cardiol. 1988 Dec;12 (6 Suppl A): 3A-13A.
4 Van DeWerf, F. and Baim, D.S. Reperfusion for ST-segment elevation myocardial infarction: An overview of current treatment options. Circulation 2002; 105: 2813. http://circ.ahajournals.org/cgi/content/full/circulationaha;105/24/2813

Review

Level 1: Content knowledge

1 Which of the following statements describes the cardiovascular response normally seen in cardiogenic shock?
   A Right ventricular end-diastolic volume decreased, cardiac output decreased, systemic vascular resistance increased
   B Right ventricular end-diastolic volume increased, cardiac output decreased, systemic vascular resistance increased
   C Right ventricular end-diastolic volume decreased, cardiac output decreased, systemic vascular resistance decreased
   D Right ventricular end-diastolic volume increased, cardiac output decreased, systemic vascular resistance decreased

2 Acidosis is often seen in the later stages of shock. Which of the following statements is *not* true?
   A Impaired kidney function prevents adequate excretion of excess hydrogen ions.
   B Decreased oxygen delivery to the cells increases the production of lactic acid that contributes to the development of an acidosis.
   C Acidosis stimulates heart activity offsetting, to some degree, the reduction in tissue perfusion seen in shock.
   D Acidosis reduces the reactivity of resistance vessels to neurally released catecholamines.

3 A patient suffering from which type of shock will have the lowest increase in blood pressure with infusion of 1 L of normal saline?
   A Haemorrhagic shock
   B Cardiogenic shock
   C Distributive
   D Obstructive

Level 2: Clinical applications

1 Which of the following therapies has the strongest evidence to support its use in cardiac arrest?
   A Closed chest compressions
   B Intravenous adrenaline
   C Defibrillation
   D Intubation and ventilation
   E Intravenous amiodarone

107

2   Which of the following clinical situations is most likely to result in a successful resuscitation?

A   An 89-year-old male found not breathing and pulseless; ambulance called and 10 minutes later the rhythm strip shows asystole.

B   A 46-year-old female collapses and receives basic life support immediately, and when the paramedics arrive her initial rhythm is ventricular fibrillation.

C   A 39-year-old male is found collapsed in his car, and after 10 minutes (with no CPR) the ambulance arrive to find him pulseless and in fine ventricular fibrillation.

D   A 22-year-old male driver of a motor vehicle is injured in a high speed crash; he is in cardiac arrest when the ambulance arrives and CPR commences.

E   A 73-year-old male complains of chest pain; his initial ECG shows a large anterior myocardial infarction. He arrests, and his rhythm is pulseless electrical activity .

3   Which of the following ECG findings are not indications for consideration of reperfusion therapy?

A   2 mm ST elevation in leads II, III and aVF

B   New left bundle branch block

C   1 mm ST elevation in leads V2–5

D   T-wave inversion in leads V2–5

E   2 mm ST elevation in leads II, III and aVF with ST depression in leads V1–2

Level 3: Topics for further discussion

1   Discuss the 'chain of survival' and how systems and various interventions can improve survival from cardiac arrest.

2   Review the evidence surrounding advanced cardiac life support.

Case 8
Holly was struggling to get her breath ...

An 8-year-old girl is rushed to the Emergency Department with history of shortness of breath since last night; she is breathless, agitated, and has an audible wheeze. You need to act quickly to stabilise her and prevent further deterioration.

Timeline summary

22:00	Shortness of breath; salbutamol administered by spacer device at home.
01:00–05:00	Salbutamol administered hourly.
05:00	Wheeze is more pronounced; drowsy and unable to speak.
05:15	Presents to the Emergency Department.
05:15–05:35	Initial management.
05:35	Escalation of therapy; arterial blood gas (ABG) taken; addition of intravenous salbutamol and inhaled ipratropium bromide.
06:00	Slow response to therapy; add magnesium sulfate.
06:30	Improved clinical state; referred to intensive care unit (ICU); continuing therapy.
07:45	Transferred to ICU.

Learning objectives

Physiological

- Understand how obstructive and restrictive patterns of airway disease differ.
- Describe how airways resistance affects ventilation and blood gases.
- Understand how the physiological mechanisms of airway narrowing cause the resulting signs and respiratory distress.

Clinical

- Understand the fundamentals of the emergency management of acute asthma.
- Describe the long-term issues surrounding asthma treatment and the role of a well-developed management plan.
- Be able to describe and classify the severity of an acute episode of asthma.

Context

Holly was diagnosed with asthma when she was 4 years old. She would get wheezy and breathless whenever she developed an upper respiratory tract infection. She was well and active in between exacerbations, and used salbutamol only as required. She is otherwise in excellent health and enjoys participating in sports and outdoor activities. She suffers from hay fever, as does her older sister.

It is currently mid-winter and there has been a lot of smoke in the atmosphere from wood heaters. Holly has had a dry cough and a sore throat for the last two days, but she has not been wheezy or particularly breathless. Her mother has been watching her carefully, and administered salbutamol by a spacer device when she became more breathless in the early evening. She settled well, and went to bed at 8:00 p.m.

22:00 hours

Holly woke up coughing, with a marked wheeze. Her mother again administered 6 puffs of salbutamol via the spacer, with a good effect. Holly went back to bed, her wheeze having settled.

01:00–05:00 hours

Holly awoke a number of times throughout the night, and had similar doses of salbutamol each hour. However, her wheeze never completely responded to therapy and her parents became concerned because she had never had an attack quite this bad.

05:00 hours

Holly's wheeze suddenly became more pronounced. She couldn't speak more than a few words, she couldn't stop coughing and she became drowsy. Her parents recognised that she was becoming increasingly unwell and they rapidly drove to the Emergency Department at the local hospital.

Clinical question 1

(a) Discuss the initial presentation and treatment of Holly's asthma.
(b) Classify this exacerbation as mild, moderate or severe based upon the clinical features above.

05:15 hours

You are a junior doctor on duty in Emergency Department, when Holly is carried in by her parents. She is agitated and appears to be blue around her lips. She has an audible wheeze, and can speak only a few words at a time in response to questions.

The nurse in the resuscitation bay rapidly administers 10 L/min oxygen via a mask and you place your stethoscope onto her chest. There is some air entry, but it sounds quieter than you expect.

Clinical comment

A steady deterioration has been described, with precipitants most likely being the combination of infectious and environmental agents.

Holly has a number of features indicating a life-threatening exacerbation of asthma, as defined by the National Asthma Council of Australia. She is drowsy, is too breathless to speak, and appears to have central cyanosis. This is clearly a medical emergency and requires a rapid and effective response.

Recognising a life-threatening asthma attack you call both the emergency and paediatric registrars and commence treatment.

Clinical question 2

(a) Describe your initial actions when confronted with a child like this.
(b) What are your management priorities?
(c) What clinical signs would you look for to identify respiratory distress?
(d) Discuss the features that indicate that this is a severe attack of asthma.

The emergency registrar has come to your assistance and the nursing staff have administered cardiac and oxygen saturation monitoring and taken an initial set of observations:

- PR: 180 bpm
- RR: 50 breaths/min
- SpO$_2$:   92% (on 10 L/min O$_2$)
- temperature: 37.7°C
- cool peripheries, capillary refill 3 seconds

You note that she has a marked tracheal tug and that she has significant intercostal recession with inspiration. You consider obtaining a peak expiratory flow reading, but quickly realise she is too sick for such a task.

A nebuliser mask is applied and 5 mg of salbutamol is immediately administered. Intravenous access is obtained, and you administer 1 mg/kg of intravenous methylprednisolone. You obtain a brief history from her parents.

Clinical question 3

(a) How will you clinically assess Holly's response to therapy? Use this opportunity to review resuscitation protocols for children.
(b) Medication and fluid is administered on a 'per kilogram' basis in children. How do you estimate weight in children?

Clinical comment

Whenever confronted with a seriously ill patient, assessment and management occur in parallel. Resuscitation begins immediately, and senior help is summoned. Initial management is directed towards providing adequate oxygenation and treating the bronchospasm. This can occur with high-flow oxygen delivered by a mask, and by salbutamol delivered constantly by a nebuliser. Intravenous access has been obtained so that intravenous medication and fluids can be administered.

The clinical features of respiratory distress include the use of the accessory muscles of respiration during inspiration, intercostal recession during inspiration (that is, the indrawing of skin between the ribs), an inability to speak and an altered mental state. These features contribute to the classification of this being a life-threatening attack of asthma, in addition to the following: she was cyanosed upon arrival (which suggests significant hypoxia), and her vital signs reveal a tachycardia and oxygen saturations of 92% despite high-flow oxygen. Response to therapy will be judged by an improvement in these parameters and an improvement in mental state.

It is important to administer appropriate doses of medication and fluid to children. However, it is not always possible to obtain an accurate weight, especially in a situation such as this.

Some useful formulas that may help in resuscitation include:

weight = (2 × age) + 9 (under the age of 9 years)
endotracheal tube size = age/4 + 4
initial fluid bolus = 10 mL/kg

It is essential that you check the doses and formulas in use at your institution.

Using the formula to calculate Holly's weight you estimate her weight to be 25 kg. She receives 25 mg of intravenous methylprednisolone and the nebulised salbutamol continues. An intravenous bolus of 250 mL (10 mL/kg) of 0.9% normal saline is given.

05:35 hours

The air entry into Holly's lungs seems to have improved. However, she remains agitated, tachycardic and tachypnoeic. She continues to receive continuous nebulised salbutamol. You assess that she has had a minimal response to therapy and decide that additional therapy is required.

Clinical question 4

What additional therapy could you use now? Relate your answer to commonly used guidelines.

In keeping with asthma management guidelines, you administer 125 μg (5 μg/kg) of intravenous salbutamol. You also add 250 μg of ipratropium bromide to the nebuliser solution.

You take an arterial blood sample to better assess oxygenation and ventilation.

The ABG results are shown in Table 8.1.

Table 8.1 Arterial blood gas results

FIO$_2$	~0.40
Blood gas values:	
pH	7.31
PaCO$_2$	51.4 mmHg
PaO$_2$	78 mmHg
Base excess	−4.8 mmol/L
HCO$_3^-$	21.6 mmol/L
Oximetry values:	
Hb	147 g/L
SaO$_2$	94.3%
Electrolyte values:	
K$^+$	3.1 mmol/L
Na$^+$	136 mmol/L

Clinical question 5

(a) Comment upon the ABG results.

(b) How would you assess her response to therapy now?

Clinical comment

It is appropriate to increase the therapy, and intravenous salbutamol is commonly used in severe attacks. Ipratropium bromide has been added to the nebuliser solution. The ABG results reveal impaired ventilation (as evidenced by a raised PaCO$_2$) and reduced gas exchange (with a PaO$_2$ of only 78 mmHg despite an FIO$_2$ of 0.4). The main concern from a clinical perspective is whether Holly is able to maintain her conscious state and keep breathing until the therapy takes effect. She is at risk of suffering a respiratory arrest, so she must be monitored constantly and aggressive therapy must continue. The treating team must be prepared to intubate her and initiate mechanical ventilation should her condition further deteriorate—but this is dangerous in its own right, and is best avoided if at all possible. Holly does not yet appear to be at this stage.

Physiology comment

During an asthma attack the main physiological abnormality is airway obstruction (high airway resistance, leading to reduced expiratory and inspiratory flows) due to a combination of smooth muscle contraction (bronchoconstriction), inflammation of the airway wall and mucus plugging. Clinical features include wheeze, chest tightness and dyspnoea. The increased resistance to breathing can lead to hyperinflation (abnormally large total lung capacity (TLC)). An important feature of asthma, which helps to distinguish it from other diseases that cause airway obstruction, notably chronic obstructive pulmonary disease (COPD), is that it is usually intermittent and lung function often returns to normal or near normal between attacks. However, patients who have recurrent attacks (chronic asthmatics) can develop persistent airway obstruction with incomplete reversibility to bronchodilator therapy.

Airway obstruction

Airway obstruction is defined as abnormally low expiratory flows and is detected and quantified by performing spirometry. The spirometry test is performed by having the patient inspire fully (to TLC), and then to completely expire with maximal effort. The results of spirometry can be displayed either as a plot of expired volume against time (spirogram), or as plot of expired flow against volume (flow–volume curve).

The common features of airway obstruction are reductions in FEV_1, FEV_1/FVC ratio, PEF and a concavity in the descending limb of the expiratory flow–volume curve (Fig. 8.1). In more severe cases the FVC is also reduced because during the expiration the already narrowed airways close prematurely, trapping gas in the lungs and resulting in a raised residual volume (RV). If the airways are sufficiently narrowed during an asthmatic attack, the functional residual capacity (FRC) can increase as each successive expiration is prematurely interrupted by the next. An elevated FRC is often referred to as functional hyperinflation and is sometimes associated with an increase in TLC, although it is usually less than the increase in FRC.

In the emergency setting it is not always easy to obtain spirometry in distressed patients with significant airway obstruction, but if it can be obtained the results help to assess the severity of the attack and subsequently the effectiveness of therapy. Under these conditions it is often easier to obtain a measurement of PEF as this test requires the patient

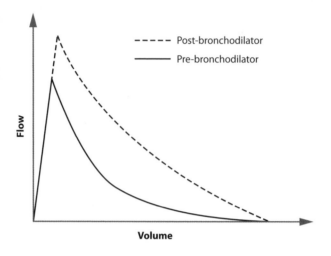

Figure 8.1 Flow–volume curve

only to blow maximally (from TLC) for a couple of seconds. Peak expiratory flow can then be used to grade severity, particularly in children and young adults where other causes of airway obstruction such as COPD are unlikely, and to monitor progression and response to therapy.

Holly had difficulty talking in complete sentences, indicating severely reduced ventilatory capacity; this is an important indicator that if the attack continues to worsen it could become life-threatening. For this reason saturated oxygen level was monitored continuously in the Emergency Department with a pulse oximeter. If the patient became hypoxaemic, oxygen would be administered simultaneously with nebulised bronchodilators. The substantially increased airway resistance can severely impair the patient's capacity to flush carbon dioxide from the lungs (that is, impair alveolar ventilation), resulting in an increase in $PaCO_2$.

06:00 hours

The blood gas results have confirmed your clinical assessment of impaired ventilation, and you anxiously wait for the inhaled and intravenous therapy to take effect.

However, Holly continues to struggle to breathe despite the aggressive therapy. You decide to add magnesium sulfate to the nebuliser.

Physiology comment

Reversibility of airway obstruction

In asthma, particularly in young people and adults who have never smoked, the degree of airway obstruction is usually reversible either spontaneously or following bronchodilator therapy. Therefore, spirometry is usually performed both before and 10–15 minutes after the administration of a bronchodilator, e.g. salbutamol. Generally, an improvement in FEV_1 of $\geq$ 12% and $\geq$ 200 mL indicates a positive response, and an improvement back to normal spirometry is strongly indicative of asthma. The shape of the flow–volume curve also improves with reduction in the depth of the concavity in the descending limb (see Fig. 8.1). After several doses of nebulised salbutamol, Holly improved, indicating dilatation of the airways and some return of ventilatory function. Although spirometry and PEF were not measured in this patient, it is certain that her FEV_1 and FEV_1/FVC ratio had improved.

Variability of lung function

With reversible disease, variability of ventilatory function (FEV_1, PEF, FEV_1/FVC)—often with spontaneous recovery to normal or near-normal values between attacks—is an important feature that is used to confirm the diagnosis. The degree of variability is commonly measured from serial measurements of PEF, obtained by having the patient record their own PEF three or four times during the day and evening for several days or weeks (see Fig. 8.2). Typically, PEF is lowest in the early morning and is referred to as 'morning dipping'. Effective treatment (such as corticosteroids) will not only reduce the within-day variability of PEF, but will increase the mean value towards normal.

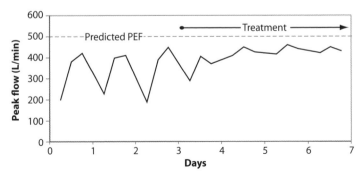

Figure 8.2 Peak flow measurements before and during treatment

06:30 hours

Holly is looking more alert, and her breathing has improved. She is now able to talk in short sentences. However, you recognise that there is still potential for deterioration. She has been awake all night struggling to breathe, and you are concerned that she may yet lose her respiratory drive due to exhaustion. You refer her for admission to the Intensive Care Unit (ICU) for continuing close monitoring and intensive treatment.

Physiology comment

Obstructive versus restrictive

The two main classifications of abnormal ventilatory function are:

- obstructive ventilatory defect. Airflow obstruction (or airflow limitation) is the most commonly seen lung function defect and is a feature of diseases such as asthma and COPD. It is characterised by difficulty blowing out quickly (that is, increased airway resistance). Thus, the features of an obstructive ventilatory defect are a reduction in all expiratory flows including FEV_1, the FEV_1/FVC ratio and PEF. As mentioned above, although spirometry was not measured in this case it is almost certain that Holly had a severe obstructive defect and the goal with therapy is to reduce the degree of obstruction.

- restrictive ventilatory defect. A restrictive ventilatory defect is characterised by loss of lung volume in the absence of airflow obstruction. Typically, the FVC is reduced, but the airway resistance is not increased and the FEV_1/FVC ratio is normal or high, indicating that there is no difficulty blowing out quickly. A restrictive ventilatory defect can be due to pulmonary (for example, interstitial lung diseases such as fibrosing alveolitis) or extra-pulmonary (for example, stiff chest wall, reduced respiratory muscle strength) factors that limit lung expansion.

07:45 hours

Holly is transferred to the ICU. She has received constant salbutamol via nebuliser and by intravenous infusion for the last 2 hours, and is now clinically much improved.

Epilogue

Holly responded well to therapy and was able to be weaned off the salbutamol infusion later in the morning. She started using her spacer again, and early the next day was transferred to the ward.

She was discharged 2 days later on a reducing dose of oral prednisolone with a revised asthma management plan that included the early use of inhaled preventer medication.

Clinical comment

Holly suffered a life-threatening asthma attack, most likely precipitated by a viral upper respiratory tract infection and the environmental influence of wood smoke. These are common triggers for asthma. Early recognition of such precipitants should activate an asthma management plan, which could include the use of either inhaled or oral corticosteroids to help prevent such exacerbations. Use of a peak flow meter can guide therapy in the home, but often children are not able to use them when they are acutely unwell. A well-described management plan developed in consultation with the family doctor is essential for any asthmatic, and can prevent such serious exacerbations.

Physiology comment

During an asthma attack the increased airway resistance is caused by airway narrowing that is brought about by constriction of airway smooth muscle (bronchoconstriction), airway inflammation and mucus plugging. This combination of events results in reduced expiratory and, to some extent, inspiratory flows at all lung volumes. Hyperinflation can occur because narrowed, small airways close prematurely or take too long to 'empty' during tidal breathing; this is compounded by a high respiratory rate. Hyperinflation can have a positive effect on airway calibre as it imposes greater traction forces on the small airways, helping to hold them open. However, this is to some extent offset due to the increased work of breathing that may result in respiratory muscle fatigue and distress. During an attack the peripheral pulse may appear to disappear (pulsus paradoxicus) during inspiration. Indicators of a severe attack requiring urgent treatment include the inability to speak in complete sentences, cyanosis, tachycardia and pulsus paradoxicus.

During an asthma attack, the degree of airway narrowing/closure is not uniform across all airways and some gas exchange regions of the lung receive little, if any, ventilation. Although some compensatory redistribution of blood flow away from the poorly ventilated regions does occur, this may be inadequate with these units still receiving significant blood flow relative to ventilation, resulting in ventilation and perfusion inequality. This causes a widening of the alveolar–arterial oxygen gradient and reduced arterial oxygenation (hypoxaemia). A further decrease in arterial oxygenation may be seen following the administration of bronchodilators despite a reduction in airway resistance, and is usually attributed to further increases in blood flow to poorly ventilated units. A decrease in $PaCO_2$ is commonly seen during a mild attack or in the early phase of an attack due to overall high alveolar ventilation (hyperventilation), presumably due to hypoxic stimulation of ventilation as well as anxiety. However, an abnormally high $PaCO_2$ (and fall in pH), as was observed in Holly's case, is a serious sign and a clear indication of life-threatening asthma due to respiratory muscle fatigue and incipient respiratory failure.

References and further reading

1 Blitz, M., Blitz, S., Beasely, R., Diner, B.M., Hughes, R., Knopp, J.A., Rowe, B.H. Inhaled magnesium sulfate in the treatment of acute asthma. The Cochrane Database of Systematic Reviews 2005; Issue 3.
2 Plotnick, L.H., Ducharme, F.M. Combined inhaled anticholinergics and beta2-agonists for initial treatment of acute asthma in children. The Cochrane Database of Systematic Reviews 2000; Issue 3.
3 National Asthma Council Australia. *Asthma Management Handbook 2002.* South Melbourne, National Asthma Council Australia. www.nationalasthma.org.au (severity classification and treatment, pp. 29–30)
4 Paediatric resuscitation guidelines. Australian Resuscitation Council. www.resus.org.au
5 Review of paediatric life support algorithms and policies at the American Heart Association. www.americanheart.org/presenter.jhtml?identifier=3026175
6 Smith, M., Iqbal, S., Elliott, T.M., Rowe, B.H. Corticosteroids for hospitalised children with acute asthma. The Cochrane Database of Systematic Reviews 2003; Issue 1.

Review

Level 1: Content knowledge

1 The effort-independent portion of the forced vital capacity manoeuvre (FVC) consists of which of the following?
   A First 20% to 30% of the FVC manoeuvre
   B Last 70% to 80% of the FVC manoeuvre
   C Middle portion of the FVC manoeuvre
   D First 50% of the FVC manoeuvre
   E Entire forced vital capacity manoeuvre
2 Which of the following may occur in patients suffering from extrinsic asthma?
   A Bronchi hyperreactive to common stimuli
   B Excess mucus secretion in the bronchioles
   C Increased histamine release from mast cells
   D All of the above
3 Corticosteroids can be useful in asthma management as they:
   A Reduce bronchial hyperreactivity
   B Dilate narrowed bronchioles
   C Increase bronchial hyperreactivity
   D Prevent the release of type II alveolar cell mediators

Level 2: Clinical applications

1 Which of the following therapies are *not* indicated for the management of a severe exacerbation of asthma?
   A Constant salbutamol by nebuliser
   B Administration of a systemic corticosteroid
   C Titration of oxygen saturations to less than 92%
   D Magnesium chloride by nebuliser or intravenous use
   E Nebulised adrenaline
2 Match the following clinical presentations of asthma with the appropriate clinical classification:
   A Laboured respirations, speaking in words only, PEF < 40% predicted
   B Exertional symptoms, able to speak normally, PEF > 60% predicted
   C Exhausted and confused, cyanosed, unable to speak
   D Dyspnoea at rest, wheeze, able to speak short sentences, PEF 40–60% predicted
      (i) Mild
      (ii) Moderate
      (iii) Severe
      (iv) Life-threatening

3 Which of the following bedside observations or investigations would you *not* expect in a patient with a moderate exacerbation of asthma?
A Widespread audible expiratory wheeze
B Oxygen saturations > 94% on room air
C PEFR > 400 L/min
D Pulse rate of 100
E Respiratory rate of 24

Level 3: Topics for further discussion

1 Describe the need for a written management plan to be provided when patients with asthma are discharged from Emergency Departments.
2 Discuss other interventions that may be of use when managing a patient with severe asthma.

Case 9
Mr Hanlon couldn't breathe ...

A breathless 75-year-old patient presents to the Emergency Department barely breathing and with a reduced conscious state. Your clinical skills combined with a working knowledge of respiratory physiology will lead to the optimal management of this man. A series of arterial blood gas results demonstrate the appropriate use of this diagnostic test.

Timeline summary

16:10	Presents to Emergency Department.
16:20	Arterial blood gas (ABG) sample taken.
16:30	Bilevel positive airway pressure (BiPAP); continuation of assessment and management.
16:40	Intravenous access is obtained, bloods are taken, commence treatment of severe infective exacerbation of emphysema.
16:45	Chest X-ray (CXR) obtained.
17:30	Repeat ABG obtained.
19:00	Third ABG obtained.
20:40	Fourth ABG obtained.

Learning objectives

Physiological

- Describe the difference between type 1 and type 2 respiratory failure.
- Understand the basic physiology of blood gases.
- Define the physiological determinants of $PaCO_2$.
- Understand how $PaCO_2$ can become elevated in patients suffering from chronic obstructive pulmonary disease (COPD).

- Describe the physiological basis of using assisted ventilation when treating COPD.

Clinical

- Understand the clinical difference between gas exchange and ventilation.
- Be able to recognise inadequate ventilation in an ill patient.
- In conjunction with clinical signs, be able to utilise the ABG to track improvements or deterioration in a patient's condition.
- Understand the basic concepts of non-invasive ventilation.

Context

Mr Hanlon is a 75-year-old male who lives at home with his wife. He is a retired plumber, and has smoked heavily for the last 60 years. He 'gets around all right' but has been becoming more breathless over the last 2 years. His family doctor diagnosed him with emphysema 12 months ago, after taking a history and performing a CXR (Fig. 9.1).

At the time, he was advised to stop smoking and therapy was commenced, consistent with COPD clinical practice guidelines. Smoking cessation was partially successful, but after smoking for such a long time, he found it incredibly hard to give up. He used his salbutamol puffer regularly.

Clinical question 1

How do you interpret the CXR?

Clinical comment

The CXR shows hyperinflated lung fields, indicating widespread alveolar damage consistent with chronic obstructive pulmonary disease. Put simply, there is more 'black' where there should be the 'white' of healthy lung tissue.

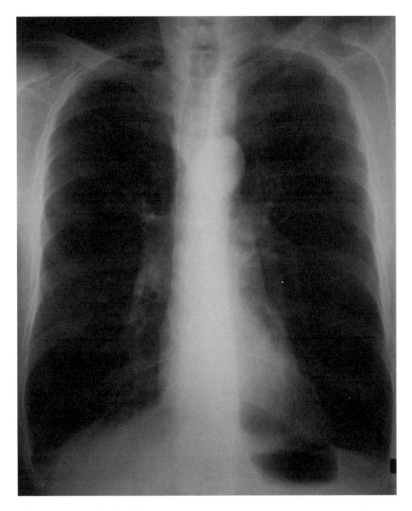

Figure 9.1 Initial chest X-ray

At the time of diagnosis, he was also referred to a respiratory physician who performed respiratory function tests (RFTs) and analysis of arterial blood (see Table 9.1).

Table 9.1 Respiratory function and arterial blood gas test results

	Pre-bronchodilator		
	Actual	**Predicted**	**% Predicted**
Spirometry:			
FEV_1 (L)	0.64	3.03	21.1
FVC (L)	1.96	3.98	49.2
FEV_1/FVC (%)	32	76	
$FEF_{25-75\%}$ (L/s)	0.27	3.04	8.9
PEF (L/s)	3.16	7.92	39.9
Arterial gases:			
Inspired O_2 (%)	21.00		
pH	7.40	7.40	
$PaCO_2$ (mmHg)	50.0	38–42	
PaO_2 (mmHg)	71.0	78.0	
HCO_3 (mmol/L)	30.9	24	
BE (mmol/L)	5.0		
$P(A-a)O_2$ (mmHg)	18.6		
Hb (gm/dL)	12.9	12–18	
SaO_2 (%)	95.1		
COHb (%)	3.4	<1.5 %	

Clinical question 2

(a) How do you interpret the RFTs?
(b) What therapy would you commence?

Clinical comment

The respiratory function tests indicate an obstructive pattern: the FEV_1/ FVC ratio is low. The arterial blood gas results reveal a compensated chronic respiratory alkalosis: the partial pressure of carbon dioxide ($PaCO_2$) is elevated at 50 mmHg and the bicarbonate has increased to 30.9 mmol/L, indicating metabolic compensation, producing the net effect of a normal pH.

Having Confirmed the diagnosis and assessed the severity, management should be consistent with the principles as outlined in the COPDX plan:

- **O**ptimise function.
- **P**revent deteriorations.
- **D**evelop support network and self-management plan.
- **M**anage e**X**acerbations.

Two days ago Mr Hanlon developed a mild cough, which was productive with green sputum. He usually had a cough, so didn't take too much notice. He used his salbutamol more regularly, but nevertheless found himself becoming increasingly out of breath and unable to even get up. He had hardly slept last night, and this morning was finding it increasingly hard to breathe. His wife found him semi-conscious in his chair and called the ambulance.

16:10 hours

Mr Hanlon has just arrived in the Emergency Department and is semi-conscious ...

Your first thought is that he looks extremely sick. He is only just breathing, is grey and sweaty, and you listen to his chest and hear ... nothing.

Clinical question 3

(a) How will you manage him immediately?
(b) What interventions are available and/or appropriate?

16:20 hours

Oxygen is continued, monitoring is applied, and you decide to take an arterial blood sample to confirm your suspicions.

Clinical question 4

What do you expect the ABG to reveal?

Table 9.2 Arterial blood gas results

FIO$_2$	0.5
Blood gas values:	
pH	7.142
PaCO$_2$	127 mmHg
PaO$_2$	42.2 mmHg
BE	7.1 mmol/L
HCO$_3^-$	41.6 mmol/L
Oximetry values:	
Hb	141g/L
SaO$_2$	69.2%
Hct	43.3%
Electrolyte values:	
K$^+$	5.1 mmol/L
Na$^+$	141 mmol/L
Ca$^+$	1.35 mmol/L
Metabolite values:	
Glu	6.7 mmol/L
Lac	0.5 mmol/L

Physiology comment

Blood gases

The uptake of oxygen and elimination of carbon dioxide (gas exchange) and the control of arterial oxygen and carbon dioxide tensions are the cardinal functions of the respiratory system. The arterialisation of mixed venous blood occurs through passive diffusion across the lung membrane and is fairly well understood. However, the control of blood gas tensions is the result of a complex feedback system involving special structures and circuits that are less well understood, but are remarkably well designed to rapidly adjust ventilation to meet the body's varying demands.

In health and at sea level the PaCO$_2$ is normally maintained at about 40 mmHg and PaO$_2$ at between 80 and 100 mmHg, depending on age. Respiratory failure is defined by hypoxaemia (low arterial oxygen tension; <60 mmHg) in the presence of either a normal PaCO$_2$ (type 1) or an elevated PaCO$_2$ (type 2). Type 2 respiratory failure is seen in patients with respiratory diseases such as COPD, particularly during an acute exacerbation.

The $PaCO_2$ of arterial blood is inversely related to the degree of alveolar ventilation; that is, if ventilation is doubled, $PaCO_2$ is halved (hyperventilation). The reduction in $PaCO_2$ due to hyperventilation results in an elevation of the alveolar PO_2 (PAO_2) and hence PaO_2. This is described by the alveolar–air equation:

$$PaO_2 \approx PAO_2 = PIO_2 - PaCO_2/0.8$$

where PIO_2 is the partial pressure of inspired oxygen (at sea level, PIO_2 = (Pb – 47) × 0.21), 0.8 is the volumetric ratio of carbon dioxide entering the alveoli to oxygen leaving the alveoli (that is, the respiratory exchange ratio) and is often assumed to be 0.8 at rest. This equation can be used to quantify the effect of a reduction in $PaCO_2$ (that is, hypoventilation) or rise in $PaCO_2$ (that is, hyperventilation) on PAO_2.

The maintenance of physiological $PaCO_2$, PaO_2 (and pH) tensions is achieved by neuronal units called chemoreceptors, which regulate ventilation via the central respiratory regulator located in the floor of the brain. Normally, the level of ventilation is set by medullary chemoreceptors to maintain a $PaCO_2$ of 40 mmHg. However, if PaO_2 falls to below about 60 mmHg (hypoxaemia), ventilation is stimulated by peripheral chemoreceptors (aortic and carotid bodies) that serve to elevate PaO_2 as described by the alveolar–air equation above.

Clinical question 5

(a) Interpret the ABG results. Consider the $P(A\text{-}a)O_2$ gradient and the acid–base status.

(b) What therapy would be worth trying *right now*?

Clinical comment

Mr Hanlon is seriously ill and in type 2 respiratory failure. Despite the administration of oxygen he is markedly hypoxaemic, and with a $PaCO_2$ of 127 mmHg it is quite apparent that he is hardly breathing and has a marked acute or chronic respiratory acidosis. This result was to be expected, as clinically he was obtunded due to his breathing being insufficient. The PaO_2 of 42.2 mmHg indicates significant hypoxaemia, especially considering that the patient is receiving 50% oxygen by mask. The alveolar gas equation confirms the A-a gradient to be nearly 200 mmHg.

129

He needs urgent ventilatory support and, given his reasonable quality of life beforehand, it seems appropriate to initiate therapy. There are two options available: invasive ventilation and non-invasive ventilation. While a decision is being made as to which therapy to offer, his airway can be supported and his breathing can be enhanced by the use of a bag-valve-mask device.

16:30 hours

The BiPAP machine is rapidly brought to the bedside and a tight-fitting mask is placed on the patient (see Fig. 9.2).

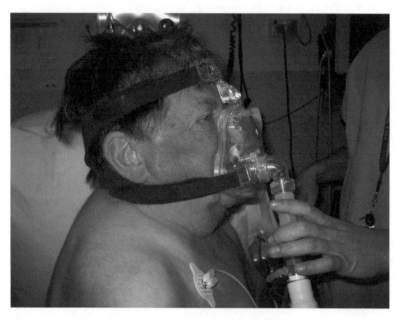

Figure 9.2 Non-invasive ventilation (NIV) mask being fitted on patient

The controls are set as follows:

- inspiratory positive airway pressure (IPAP): 12 mmHg
- expiratory positive airway pressure (EPAP): 5 mmHg
- FIO_2: 0.8

Physiology comment

In lung conditions such as COPD, the $PaCO_2$ can become chronically elevated (hypercapnia) due to reduced sensitivity of the medullary chemoreceptors, and the stimulus for ventilation then comes from hypoxic stimulation of the peripheral chemoreceptor. In an exacerbation of COPD, the PaO_2 can fall to dangerously low levels and it is necessary to administer supplementary oxygen. This increases the PaO_2, but can inadvertently remove or reduce the hypoxic stimulus to breathe. This results in a fall in ventilation (hypoventilation), leading to an elevation in $PaCO_2$, which can reach life-threatening levels.

It is therefore critical to monitor $PaCO_2$ and PaO_2 if supplementary oxygen is required, with the aim of administering only enough oxygen to raise the PaO_2 to an acceptable level. This may be achieved using low flow oxygen (for example, 2–3 L/min) delivered via nasal prongs or via a Venturi mask set to deliver 24–28% oxygen. Remember, these patients can have very significant airflow limitation and are usually functionally hyperinflated (that is, the lungs are over-inflated), which severely limits their capacity to maintain adequate ventilation, and any reduction in ventilatory drive is superimposed on this. Under these circumstances the patient may require supplemental ventilatory assistance to achieve adequate ventilation for the treatment of hypercapnia.

A common and very effective non-invasive method of assisting ventilation is to apply BiPAP directly to the upper airway via a tight-fitting mask. Inspiration is assisted by applying a positive airway pressure (IPAP) to the mask, and expiration is assisted by applying a lower airway pressure (EPAP) to the mask to prevent the lung airways from collapsing. In dangerously ill patients who are unable to tolerate BiPAP, mechanical ventilation via endotracheal intubation is indicated.

You start BiPAP and continue Mr Hanlon's assessment and management.

Clinical question 6

(a) What exactly is BiPAP?
(b) How would you assess his response to this therapy?
(c) What would you do now?

16:40 hours

IV access is obtained and bloods are taken. You suspect Mr Hanlon has a severe infective exacerbation of his emphysema and, in keeping with established management guidelines, the following treatment is administered:

- intravenous corticosteroid: hydrocortisone 200 mg
- constant nebulised salbutamol 5 mg via the BiPAP circuit
- 1 g intravenous ceftriaxone and 300 mg oral roxithromycin.

16:45 hours

Following commencement of treatment, a mobile CXR is rapidly obtained (see Fig. 9.3).

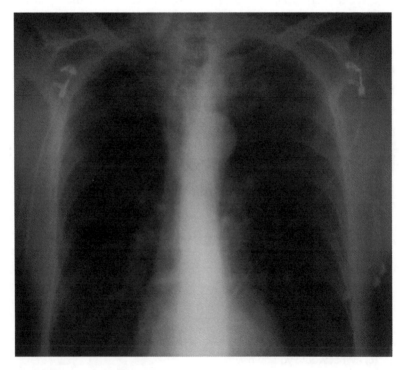

Figure 9.3 Second chest X-ray

Clinical question 7

Comment on the CXR. What specific features would you be looking for in this case?

Clinical comment

The clinical findings consistent with COPD are expected, but the CXR is performed to find causes for the acute exacerbation, such as pneumothorax, consolidation and pulmonary oedema.

17:30 hours

A repeat ABG is obtained 80 minutes after Mr Hanlon's arrival (see Table 9.3).

Table 9.3 Second arterial blood gas results

FIO_2	0.4
pH	7.227
$PaCO_2$	99.6 mmHg
PaO_2	45.3 mmHg
BE	8.3 mmol/L
HCO_3^-	39.9 mmol/L

Clinical question 8

(a) How do these values compare to the previous reading?
(b) Do you think the situation is improving?
(c) What is the role of oxygen in respiratory failure in COPD?

Mr Hanlon's condition seems to be improving. He seems to be moving more air into his lungs and he is looking more alert, but is still quite unwell. You decide to continue with the BiPAP therapy and to re-assess him continually.

19:00 hours

Another ABG is obtained 90 minutes later (see Table 9.4).

Table 9.4 Fourth arterial blood gas results

FIO_2	0.4
pH	7.272
$PaCO_2$	84.3 mmHg
PaO_2	53.3 mmHg
BE	7.8 mmol/L
HCO_3^-	37.6 mmol/L

Clinical comment

BiPAP is a form of non-invasive ventilation that can be initiated easily in the Emergency Department. It can provide respiratory support to patients with respiratory failure. An increased pressure forces gas into the lungs at a set respiratory rate, causing inspiration. When the patient exhales an expiratory pressure is provided to recruit collapsed alveoli and to reduce the work of breathing. This may provide enough respiratory support to improve ventilation and avoid the need for intubation.

Consider the effect on Mr Hanlon; note that his carbon dioxide has fallen and his pH has increased, indicating that his gases are improving. However, his clinical status will predominantly guide therapy. If this is not up to a satisfactory standard (that is, he is not maintaining his airway, he becomes fatigued, his conscious state declines further, he becomes even more hypoxaemic, or he can't tolerate the tight-fitting BiPAP mask), then definitive airway management may be necessary, and he will require intubation.

Trying non-invasive ventilation (NIV) first is entirely appropriate: When comparing non-invasive and invasive ventilation in COPD patients with advanced hypercapnic acute respiratory failure, Squadrone et al. (2004) found that NIV had a high rate of failure. However, it provided some advantages compared with conventional invasive ventilation. Subgroup analysis suggested that the delay in intubation was not deleterious in the patients who failed NIV, whereas a better outcome was confirmed for the patients who avoided intubation. Oxygen should be titrated against the clinical effect in these patients. There is a risk that, in some patients who have lost the stimulatory effects of an elevated $PaCO_2$ through chronic carbon dioxide retention, excess oxygen may cause them to lose any stimulus to breathe, thereby worsening their already impaired ventilation. It is good practice to aim for oxygen saturations between 88 and 92%. Put simply, these patients do not need a PaO_2 any higher than 60 mm Hg.

20:40 hours

A bed is arranged in the High Dependency Unit (HDU) and the BiPAP continues. Mr Hanlon's mental state continues to improve and you wish to confirm his improvement in respiratory status by taking another ABG (see Table 9.5).

Table 9.5 Fifth arterial blood gas results

FIO_2	0.4
pH	7.322
$PaCO_2$	71.9 mmHg
PaO_2	45.6 mmHg
BE	8.0 mmol/L
HCO_3^-	36.1 mmol/L

This arterial blood sample was taken 4.5 hours after his arrival—his pH has almost normalised.

Clinical question 9

What do you think his normal $PaCO_2$ would be? *Hint:* look closely at his HCO_3^- level.

135

Clinical comment

The blood gases show a progressive decline in $PaCO_2$, indicating improving alveolar ventilation. The fifth ABG reveals a pH that has almost normalised, yet the $PaCO_2$ is still elevated at nearly 72 mmHg. The bicarbonate is elevated at 36 mmol/L, suggesting that he has a chronic respiratory acidosis with metabolic compensation; that is, his $PaCO_2$ is significantly elevated even between exacerbations. Treating clinicians should be aware of this so that appropriate end-points of therapy can be identified.

Mr Hanlon has made it through the first stage of his therapy; his clinical state has objectively improved and he has managed to avoid intubation. Of course, prevention would be ideal and an action plan needs to be discussed and implemented in the future, to reduce the risks of life-threatening exacerbations such as this.

Epilogue

Mr Hanlon was admitted to the HDU for 24 hours and then was discharged to the ward. After a 5-day stay in hospital he was discharged home.

References and further reading

1 Guidelines on non-invasive ventilation in acute respiratory failure: British Thoracic Society Standards of Care Committee. Thorax 2002; 57: 192–211. http://www.brit-thoracic.org.uk/docs/NIV.pdf
2 Squadrone, E., Frigerio, P., Fogliati, C., Gregoretti, C., Conti, G., Antonelli, M., Costa, R., Baiardi, P., Navalesi, P. Noninvasive vs invasive ventilation in COPD patients with severe acute respiratory failure deemed to require ventilatory assistance. Intensive Care Med. 2004 Jul; 30(7): 1303–10.
3 The COPDX Plan: Australian and New Zealand guidelines for the management of chronic obstructive pulmonary disease 2003. MJA. 2003; 178 (6 Suppl 17 Mar): S1–S40. http://www.mja.com.au/public/issues/178_06_170303/tho10508_all.html
4 Turnock, A.C., Walters, E.H., Walters, J.A.E., Wood-Baker, R. Action plans for chronic obstructive pulmonary disease. The Cochrane Database of Systematic Reviews 2005; Issue 4. Art. No.: CD005074.

Review

Level 1: Content knowledge

1 In health and at sea level the $PaCO_2$ and PaO_2 are normally maintained respectively at about:
   - A 60 mmHg and 80–100 mmHg
   - B 40 mmHg and 80–100 mmHg
   - C 30 mmHg and 80–100 mmHg
   - D 30 mmHg and 100–110 mmHg
2 The relative hypoventilation that may occur when administering oxygen therapy to patients with COPD is caused by:
   - A Increased sensitivity of the medullary chemoreceptors
   - B Reduced sensitivity of the medullary chemoreceptors
   - C Reduced sensitivity of the peripheral chemoreceptors
   - D Increased sensitivity of the peripheral chemoreceptors
3 If alveolar ventilation is doubled, the $PaCO_2$ is:
   - A Tripled
   - B Halved
   - C Doubled
   - D Not altered

Level 2: Clinical applications

1 Which of the following interventions should *not* be used in a patient presenting with an exacerbation of emphysema?
   - A Salbutamol administered by nebuliser
   - B High-flow oxygen to achieve oxygen saturations > 95%
   - C Administration of oral corticosteroid
   - D Spirometry and arterial blood gas
   - E Ipratropium administered by nebuliser
2 All of the following patients have confirmed emphysema. Match the following clinical scenarios with the most likely precipitant of exacerbation of emphysema:
   - A A 75-year-old male presents with a cough productive of green sputum and fevers over the preceding 2 days.
   - B An 80 year-old male complains of a sudden onset of sharp right-sided chest pain after coughing. He is breathless and there is decreased air entry on the right.
   - C A 67-year-old female is in hospital for an operation, and is prescribed medication to help her sleep.

D A 72-year-old female presents with increasing breathlessness and bilateral swollen ankles. Her jugular venous pressure is elevated.

E A 56-year-old male falls and injures the left side of his chest 2 days previous to examination.

  (i) Broken rib impeding ventilation leading to sputum retention

  (ii) Acute bronchitis

  (iii) Spontaneous pneumothorax due to bullae rupture

  (iv) Decreased respiratory drive due to sedative use

  (v) Acute right heart failure

3 Which of the following arterial blood gas results would you expect in a patient with an acute exacerbation of chronic emphysema? (*Note*: the FIO_2 is 0.21 in each case.)

	A	**B**	**C**	**D**	**E**	**Range**
pH	7.47	7.15	7.21	7.29	7.40	7.36–7.44
PO_2	69	55	73	54	65	80–100 mmHg
PCO_2	33	75	16	84	52	36–44 mmHg
HCO_3^-	24	26	11	36	29	24 mmol/L

Level 3: Topics for further discussion

1 Are there any additional therapies that could be utilised in the care of the patient with an acute exacerbation of COPD?

2 Discuss the role of antibiotic therapy for the treatment of these patients in your institution.

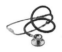

Case 10
Pete had been feeling increasingly depressed over the past few days ...

Pharmacology is physiology in action: the body's processes are modified to produce a therapeutic effect. Sometimes the therapeutic window can be narrow. The combination of mental illness and pharmaceutical products can at times be lethal. This patient presents to the Emergency Department dangerously ill, requiring specialist knowledge in physiology, resuscitation and toxicology.

Timeline summary

10:30	Pete takes an overdose of tablets.
10:50	Presents to ambulance station; transported to hospital.
11:05	Arrives at the Emergency Department; medical assessment commences.
11:12	Intravenous access, 12-lead electrocardiogram (ECG) taken.
11:19	Condition deteriorates: seizure, first arterial blood gas (ABG), preparation for intubation.
11:25–11:50	Intubation, second ECG, continuing resuscitation.
12:15	Second ABG.
12:47	Transfer to intensive care unit (ICU).

Learning objectives

Physiological

- List the four main classes of antidepressants.
- Describe the monoamine neurotransmitter deficit theory of depression.

- Understand the physiological processes occurring at the synapse and how this knowledge underpins the pharmacological treatment of depression.
- Describe the mode of action of tricyclic antidepressant (TCA) drugs.
- Describe the characteristics of anticholinergic syndrome.
- Understand the physiological basis of TCA toxicity.
- Explain the effect of TCAs on the cardiovascular system.
- Understand the physiological basis of the need to treat TCA-induced seizures aggressively.
- Describe the mechanisms by which sodium loading and blood alkalinisation are effective in treating TCA toxicity.

Clinical

- Be able to describe the principles of the initial assessment and management of the poisoned patient.
- Be able to use clinical signs and appropriate investigations to detect poisoning in patients presenting with poisoning.
- Recognise the clinical features of a serious poisoning.
- Be able to describe common toxidromes and their clinical significance.

Context

Pete had been feeling increasingly frustrated over the recent few days. He had not worked for a few months now, and the financial pressures were steadily building. He had been drinking more than usual, and his relationship with his partner of 3 years had deteriorated. It had deteriorated so much in fact that last week she walked out. Pete felt he had reached rock bottom, and he wasn't quite sure what to do next.

Medication had helped him a little over the last few months—his family doctor had prescribed him dothiepin, an antidepressant. However, he rarely had enough time to go into the details of his difficulties, and it was almost impossible to get an appointment in less than a fortnight. Pete didn't mention the drinking and the illicit drug use to his doctor.

10:30 hours

Pete feels he needed help and isn't sure how to find it. He takes a number of tablets of his antidepressant medication and walks to the local ambulance station where he calmly relays his story to the front receptionist.

'I want to kill myself. I've taken 120 of my antidepressant tablets.'

Recognising a potentially serious overdose, a paramedic crew is activated and they quickly transport him to the closest Emergency Department. He is stable throughout the journey and arrives just a little bit drowsy. His vital signs in the ambulance are as follows:

- PR: 110 bpm
- BP: 120/80 mmHg
- RR: 20 breaths/min
- GCS: 14—E3 V5 M6

Clinical question 1

(a) Describe the general principles of the initial assessment and management of the poisoned patient.
(b) Is this a serious ingestion?
(c) What clinical signs and complications would you be expecting?

11:05 hours

He is triaged 'category 2' and placed into a monitored bed in the Emergency Department. He is seen rapidly and he repeats his story to the doctor. The nursing staff set up the monitoring equipment and obtain an ECG. Intravenous access is obtained with an 18G cannula in his right antecubital fossa. The emergency physician does a rapid calculation:

'An hour ago he took 120 × 75 mg dothiepin tablets—that is 9 grams of a tricyclic antidepressant. This could be serious.'

Physiology comment

Overview of antidepressants

Affective disorders are characterised by disturbances in mood with the main classifications being depression and mania. Depression may result from a life event (reactive) or have no obvious cause (endogenous). Severe endogenous depression carries a high risk of suicide. The neurological basis of depression is poorly understood, but the best current explanation links depression with a deficit of monoamine neurotransmitters noradrenaline and serotonin (also known as 5-Ht) in the forebrain. Drugs that affect depression therefore aim to modify amine storage, release or uptake.

Antidepressants can be broadly divided into four main classes:

- tricyclics;
- selective serotonin reuptake inhibitors;
- monoamine oxidase inhibitors;
- novel compounds.

11:12 hours

The ECG is recorded and handed to the doctor (see Fig. 10.1).

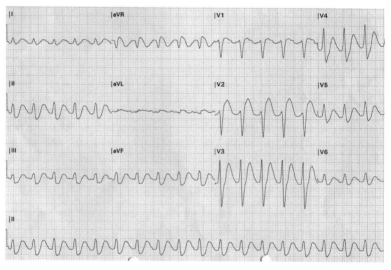

Figure 10.1 First ECG

The doctor has a closer look at the patient and notes that he is flushed, his pupils are dilated, his lips and tongue are dry, and his bowel sounds are reduced. He looks slightly drowsier than when he arrived.

Clinical question 2

(a) Interpret the ECG.

(b) Are there any concerning features?

(c) Are the clinical findings consistent with the stated ingestion?

(d) What is the name of a collection of signs and symptoms such as this?

(e) What is your risk assessment of this patient?

Clinical comment

This is a significant ingestion of a dangerous class of drug. Tricyclic antidepressants have serious side effects when ingested in quantities such as this, and this patient is already showing features of toxicity: systemic anticholinergic signs (also known as an anticholinergic 'toxidrome') and an ECG showing a tachycardia, a widened QRS interval (156 ms) and a prolonged QTc interval (491 ms). This patient is at high risk of neurological and cardiovascular complications, which are the most serious side effects of a tricyclic antidepressant overdose.

Toxidromes are collections of clinical signs that characterise ingestions of some toxic substances. The signs described in this patient indicate significant anticholinergic effects. Other toxidromes include:

Drug	Toxidrome
Organophosphates	Excess acetylcholine: small pupils, salivation, bradycardia, vomiting
Opioids	Small pupils, bradypnoea, reduced level of consciousness
Salicylates	Tinnitus, tachypnoea, mixed respiratory alkalosis and metabolic acidosis

The amount of drug ingested, the clinical features of anticholinergic poisoning, the concerning features of the ECG and a decline in his mental state all combine to produce a risk assessment that this patient is in significant danger from this overdose.

11:19 hours

Pete is looking decidedly worse. His conscious state has deteriorated to the point that his GCS is now 8. The consultant is worried:

> 'Let's move him though to the resuscitation area and prepare to intubate him.'

The nursing staff prepares the drugs and equipment for intubation, and the patient is wheeled through to the resuscitation bay while the consultant provides basic support to the patient's airway.

As the patient arrives in the resuscitation bay he begins to have a generalised seizure. Intravenous midazolam (5 mg) is immediately given. As the seizure is controlled, pre-oxygenation with 100% oxygen continues. In the meantime the resident obtains arterial blood sample (see Table 10.1).

Table 10.1 Arterial blood gas results

FIO$_2$	1.00
Blood gas values:	
pH	6.985
PaCO$_2$	33.1 mmHg
PaO$_2$	94.6 mmHg
BE	−21.5 mmol/L
HCO$_3^-$	7.5 mmol/L
Electrolyte values:	
K$^+$	4.8 mmol/L
Na$^+$	145 mmol/L
Metabolite values:	
Glu	3.6 mmol/L
Lac	3.3 mmol/L

Clinical question 3

(a) Interpret the ABG result.
(b) Is it what you expected?
(c) Describe your immediate management of the patient at this stage.

11:25 hours

The patient is intubated with thiopentone and suxamethonium. He is hyperventilated to achieve a respiratory alkalosis. A sodium bicarbonate infusion is administered to achieve a metabolic alkalosis. A repeat ECG is obtained (see Fig. 10.2)

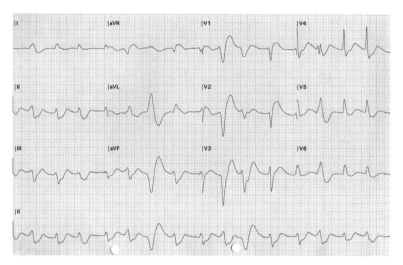

Figure 10.2 Second ECG

Clinical question 4

(a) What is the purpose of achieving an alkalosis in this patient?
(b) How would you set the ventilator?
(c) Interpret the second ECG. Comment upon the QRS and the QT intervals.

You interpret the ECG but you also refer to the machine's interpretation of the various parameters (see Table 10.2).

Table 10.2 ECG results

PR int	56 ms
QRS dur	124 ms
QT/QTc	760/642 ms

The patient is stabilised, but continues to have clinical features of anti-cholinergic poisoning. No relaxant drugs are given so that any further seizure activity can be readily recognised and treated.

12:15 hours

A repeat ABG is taken to monitor progress (see Table 10.3).

Table 10.3 Second arterial blood gas results

FIO_2	0.6
Blood gas values:	
pH	7.580
$PaCO_2$	22.6 mmHg
PaO_2	231 mmHg
HCO_3^-	21.2 mmol/L
BE	0.6 mmol/L
Electrolyte values:	
K^+	3.1 mmol/L
Na^+	135 mmol/L
Metabolite values:	
Glu	8.3 mmol/L
Lac	3.2 mmol/L

Clinical question 5

(a) Has an alkalosis been achieved?
(b) What further management is required?

12:47 hours

Pete is transferred to the ICU where he remains ventilated for two more days. A sodium bicarbonate infusion is maintained until his vital signs and ECG have normalised.

Epilogue

Pete was discharged from the ICU two days after his overdose. He was assessed by the consultation-liaison psychiatry team, who interpreted his overdose as a situational crisis. He displayed no features of major depression or psychoses, and was offered counselling and assistance to control his alcohol and illicit drug use. He was discharged from the hospital with a plan to manage his drinking and to look for employment again.

Clinical comment

This has proved to be a significant overdose with serious consequences. However, all patients with a suspected overdose should be approached using standard principles of initial assessment and management:

1 Resuscitate the patient.
2 Carry out a risk assessment.
3 Prevent absorption of the substance.
4 Enhance elimination of the substance.
5 Administer an antidote if indicated.

Resuscitation must occur promptly regardless of the cause, and standard basic life support (BLS) and advanced life support protocols apply. This extends to supportive care, whereby the patient remains intubated and closely monitored until he is capable of supporting his own airway and other vital functions.

Elements of a *risk assessment* include identification of the agent and determination of whether a clinically significant amount has been ingested. Taking an adequate and focused history is an important start, but information can be obtained from a collateral history, past history, clinical signs and the use of ancillary investigations such as the 12-lead ECG and the use of drug levels. It should be emphasised that the use of drug levels (with the exception of paracetamol) rarely influences management in the initial risk assessment of an overdose. Complications can be anticipated based upon the time of ingestion and the amount ingested. It is recommended that early advice be obtained from a clinical toxicologist, or from a commercially available toxicology database.

Prevention of absorption is an important principle of toxicological management. Activated charcoal has been adopted as the standard method of preventing absorption of many substances. The mode of action is by adsorption to the substances in the stomach, thereby preventing systemic absorption. It does not bind to lithium, heavy metals or iron. Evidence suggests that it has maximum efficacy if administered within 1 hour of ingestion.

However, there are some important issues to consider in this particular situation. Although the patient sought medical assistance promptly and met the time frame criteria for charcoal, the anticholinergic effects of TCAs upon gastrointestinal motility must be considered. The absence of bowel sounds indicates gut ileus, and failure for the charcoal to progress through the intestine may have adverse consequences such as causing a bowel obstruction.

Management of complications should follow standard clinical practice. Seizures are managed with BLS and with benzodiazepines. In addition, this patient is at significant risk of arrhythmias—despite treatment, the second ECG still has a widened QRS (>100 ms) and a markedly prolonged QT interval (760 ms). The use of specific anti-arrhythmic medications is not recommended in this situation as they may paradoxically increase the potential for arrhythmias.

Specific management of this overdose is related to manipulation of the pharmacokinetics of the medication. Plasma alkalinisation is achieved to increase the protein binding of the free drug, effectively reducing the drug available to exert its toxicity. The final arterial blood gas result indicates that an alkalosis has been achieved by both respiratory and metabolic methods. The use of cholinergic medications such as physostigmine and neostigmine to physiologically antagonise the anticholinergic effects of the ingested agent is controversial and not recommended.

Physiology comment

Physiological processes occurring at the synapse

Nerve cells (neurons) are highly specialised cells that conduct impulses throughout the central nervous system. An axon conducts impulses away from the neuronal cell body towards an effector site or connecting neuron, where it is able to release neurotransmitter chemicals. A synapse is a connection between two or more neurons or a neuron and an effector site.

When an electrical signal reaches the presynaptic terminal of a presynaptic neuron, vesicles fuse with the neuronal membrane and release their contents into the synaptic cleft. The chemicals released from the vesicles into the synaptic cleft bind to the postsynaptic receptors, producing a postsynaptic response. This response may be either stimulatory or inhibitory. A deficit of the neurotransmitters noradrenaline and serotonin has been implicated in depression. These neurotransmitters are removed from the synaptic cleft by reuptake into the presynaptic neuron (that is, they are recycled). Once back in the presynaptic neuron, the transmitters are either metabolised by the enzyme monoamine oxidase or repackaged into vesicles. Reuptake is mediated by the activity of two membrane transporter proteins, noradrenaline (NET) and serotonin (SERT). These transporters both have an approximate 200-fold selectivity for their respective neurotransmitter.

Mode of action tricyclic antidepressants

Prothiaden is a tricyclic antidepressant; its main effect is the blockade of reuptake of either noradrenaline or serotonin from the synapse back into the presynaptic terminal. Inhibition of the reuptake of either noradrenaline or serotonin, or both, appears to be associated with antidepressant activity.

Anticholinergic syndrome

The nervous system can be divided into three main systems:

- the central nervous system (CNS), consisting of the brain and spinal cord;
- the peripheral nervous system, consisting of 31 pairs of spinal nerves and 12 pairs of cranial nerves;
- the autonomic nervous system (ANS), consisting of the sympathetic and parasympathetic branches.

The ANS has two branches:

- the sympathetic division;
- the parasympathetic division.

Most organs receive input from both sympathetic and parasympathetic neurons. Commonly one branch of the autonomic nervous system will stimulate activity of an organ, whereas the other branch will inhibit activity. For example, acetylcholine (ACh) is a neurotransmitter that is released by some ANS neurons and is an excitatory neurotransmitter at some synapses (the neuromuscular junction), but inhibitory at others (cardiac pacemaker cells of the SA node). Neurons that release ACh are termed cholinergic neurons and there are two types of cholinergic receptors: nicotinic and muscarinic. Tricyclic antidepressants block muscarinic receptors via a process called anticholinergic blockade. This blockade manifests as body-wide decreased parasympathetic activity (anticholinergic syndrome), which is characterised by:

- decreased salivation and sweating;
- blurred vision;
- sinus tachycardia (see cardiovascular system effects);
- loss of GI system motility.

Toxicity of tricyclic antidepressants

The majority of the effects associated with TCA overdose result from their action as histamine, GABA-A, acetylcholine (muscarinic) and noradrenaline (α-1) receptor antagonists. Blockade of histamine receptors leads to sedation, α-receptor blockade leads to vasodilatation, GABA-A blockade may lead to seizures, and a range of anticholinergic effects result from muscarinic receptor blockade. Tricyclic antidepressants are one of the most commonly used drugs by suicide victims. Overdose of TCA primarily affects the parasympathetic nervous system (producing widespread alteration in nervous system function), cardiovascular system and CNS.

Effect of tricyclic antidepressants on the cardiovascular system

Cardiac effects

Tricyclic antidepressants alter cardiac function by three main mechanisms:

- Blockade of anticholinergic receptors causes increased heart rate and increased blood pressure (often overridden by the vascular vasodilatory effect of TCAs). Sinus tachycardia in TCA overdose is almost universal and is one of the most sensitive signs of TCA toxicity.
- Blockade of noradrenaline uptake at adrenergic presynaptic endings leads to an accumulation in the synapse and initially an increased stimulation of both central and peripheral adrenergic neurons. This increased adrenergic stimulation leads to tachycardia, increased cardiac output and hypertension (again often overridden by the vascular vasodilatory effect of TCAs). If adrenergic stimulation is pronounced it can cause ventricular ectopy and sinus tachycardia. If prolonged, norepinephrine depletion may occur and lead to decreased myocardial contractility and hypotension.
- An overdose of TCAs also blocks fast sodium channels, producing a membrane stabilising effect. This blockade acts to increase the refractory period of cardiac cells. The threshold potential is also raised, reducing cell excitability and conduction velocity through the cardiac conduction system. This may lead to a range of conduc-

tion blocks, re-entry arrhythmias and most seriously ventricular tachycardia, torsades des pointes and ventricular fibrillation.

The influx of sodium into cardiac cells initiates cardiac muscle contraction and this influx of sodium ions is responsible for the rapid upstroke of phase 0 of the cardiac muscle cell action potential. The duration of phase 0 in the heart as a whole is measured indirectly as the duration of the QRS complex on the ECG. Thus, the degree of blockade of the sodium channel can be indirectly measured by estimating QRS width. The degree of prolongation of the QRS is a reflection of TCA tissue concentrations and may be predictive of both seizures and cardiac arrhythmias.

Vascular effects

Hypotension in TCA overdose is due to a number of causes. Tricyclic antidepressants can cause direct myocardial depression, but the hypotension is usually related to α-receptor blockade induced vasodilatation. The use of α-agonists to treat the hypotension is not advisable. These inotropes can prolong the effective refractory period and thus may be pro-arrhythmic.

CNS system effects

A seizure is a convulsion caused by abnormal electrical activity in the brain. Physical manifestations of a seizure can include shaking, twitching, staring or a loss of consciousness. In TCA toxicity, the GABA-A blockade along with central anticholinergic activity have been implicated in seizure development. The central anticholinergic action of TCAs can also produce delirium and hallucinations, with many patients being comatose on admission. Although some seizures are brief, self-limiting and require no treatment, most TCA-induced seizures are treated aggressively. The acidosis produced by the seizure-induced vigorous muscle contraction and hypoxia may increase the concentration of the free drug, thereby augmenting cardiovascular toxicity.

Sodium loading and alkalinisation of blood

Tricyclic antidepressants have a broad distribution because of their highly lipophilic nature and their ability to bind proteins. In a case of overdose, diuresis and hemodialysis do not significantly increase elimination of the drug because of these properties. However, alkalinisation with sodium bicarbonate is an effective treatment as TCAs are protein-bound in an alkaline environment and therefore are less available to exert toxicity. In addition, alkalosis affects the partitioning of TCAs between the cell membrane and the sodium channel binding site, and decreases TCA-induced sodium channel blockade. Sodium loading as well as alkalinisation is effective in reversing TCA-induced conduction defects and hypotension. Sodium loading is effective as the increased extracellular concentration offsets the TCA-induced sodium channel blockade that often leads to altered cardiac function.

References and further reading

1 Blackman, K., Brown, S.G.A., Wilkes, G.J. Plasma alkalinization for tricyclic antidepressant toxicity: A systematic review. Emergency Medicine 2001; 13: 204–10.
2 Kerr, G.W., McGuffie, A.C., Wilkie, S. Tricyclic antidepressant overdose: a review. Emerg Med J 2001; 18: 236–41.
3 Mann, J.J. The medical management of depression. N Engl J Med 2005 Oct 27; 353(17): 1819–34.
4 Mokhlesi, B., Leiken, J.B., Murray. P., Corbridge, T.C. Adult toxicology in critical care: Part I: General approach to the intoxicated patient. Chest 2003; 123: 577–92.
5 Victor, W., Vieweg, R., Wood, M.A. Tricyclic antidepressants, QT interval prolongation, and torsade de pointes. Psychosomatics Sep/Oct 2004; 45(5): 371–7.

Review

Level 1: Content knowledge

1 Antidepressants can be broadly divided into which of the following main classes?
   A Tricyclics
   B Selective serotonin reuptake inhibitors
   C Monoamine oxidase inhibitors
   D Novel compounds
   E All of the above

2 Major depression is associated with:
   A A deficit of noradrenaline and serotonin in the forebrain
   B A deficit of ACh in the forebrain
   C An excess of noradrenaline and serotonin in the forebrain
   D An excess of ACh in the forebrain

3 Tricyclic antidepressants act by blockade of:
   A Reuptake of ACh from the synapse
   B Release of either noradrenaline or serotonin from the synapse
   C Release of ACh from the synapse
   D Reuptake of either noradrenaline or serotonin from the synapse

Level 2: Clinical applications

1 Match the following toxidromes with their ingestions:
   A Constricted pupils, bradypnoeic, decreased conscious state
   B Salivating, constricted pupils, sweating
   C Flushed, dry lips, large pupils, confused
   D Agitated, hypertensive, tachycardic, febrile
   E Tinnitus, metabolic acidosis and respiratory alkalosis
   (i) Salicylate poisoning
   (ii) Opioid ingestion
   (iii) Organophosphate ingestion
   (iv) Amphetamine ingestion
   (v) Anticholinergic poisoning

2 Which of the following investigations is of most use when assessing a patient with a suspected tricyclic antidepressant overdose?
   A Urinary drug screen
   B 12-lead ECG
   C Full blood count (FBC)
   D Paracetamol levels
   E All of the above are of use and influence management

3 Which is the most appropriate initial action to take when confronted with a patient with suspected poisoning?

   A Administer activated charcoal.

   B Assess airway, breathing and circulation and commence resuscitation.

   C Administer the antidote.

   D Ensure both your own and the patient's safety and summon assistance.

   E None of the above are appropriate initial actions.

4 Match the following poisons with their antidotes:

   A Paracetamol

   B Morphine

   C Iron

   D Carbon monoxide

   E Organophosphates

      (i) Oxygen

      (ii) Naloxone

      (iii) N-acetyl-cysteine

      (iv) Atropine

      (v) Desferrioxamine

5 In which of the following toxic ingestions would activated charcoal be contraindicated?

   A Iron

   B Lithium

   C Alcohol

   D Tricyclic antidepressant with absent bowel sounds

   E All of the above

6 Which of the following features would *not* be expected in an anticholinergic drug overdose?

   A Sinus tachycardia

   B Small pupils

   C Dry lips

   D Absent bowel sounds

   E Urinary retention

Level 3: Topics for further discussion

1 Discuss how to access up-to-date toxicology information when managing poisoned patients.

2 Apply the principles of toxicological management to the management of CBR (chemical, biological, radiation) incidents.

Case 11
Donna is extremely unwell after a party ...

This teenage diabetic presents to Emergency Department in the small hours of the morning with a reduced conscious state and is clinically shocked. Early diagnosis and careful emergency care are required to correct her condition. Like the previous patient, she has reduced perfusion of her vital organs—but from a different mechanism. Clinical use of the arterial blood gas results is well demonstrated in this patient.

Timeline summary

03:02	Arrives at triage in the Emergency Department and is placed on a bed in a cubicle.
03:07	Nursing assessment commences; medical staff alerted to her presence.
03:09	Medical assessment commences.
03:14	Vital signs and blood glucose level (BGL) available.
03:22	Intravenous access and bloods drawn; fluids commence; insulin infusion commences.
03:30	Arterial blood gas (ABG) sample and urine sample obtained.
03:40–05:00	Continued emergency management and referral for admission; second ABG taken.
05:00	Transfer to Intensive Care Unit (ICU)

Learning objectives

Physiological

- Understand role and function of glucose and insulin in metabolism.
- Be able to explain the physiological effects of hypoglycaemia on acid–base balance and body hydration.
- Be able to explain the physiological basis of the presenting signs of rapid breathing, significantly increased urine output, metabolic acidosis and increased BGL, as well as the presence of glucose and ketones in the urine.
- Explain why diabetic ketoacidosis (DKA) can lead to shock.

Clinical

- Recognise the features of dehydration and poor perfusion in an acutely unwell person.
- Be able to assess acid–base status using the ABG.
- Understand the clinical use of insulin, intravenous fluid and potassium in a patient with DKA.
- Describe the precipitants of DKA and the clinical approach to identifying and managing them.

Context

Donna, aged 13 years, has had type 1 diabetes for the last 3 years. She has been compliant with the diet and medication, but at times has found it frustrating. Tonight she has been staying at a friend's place, celebrating her birthday.

Donna and her friends had consumed large amounts of soft drink, chocolate and potato chips while watching movies when she reported feeling 'a bit sick' and began going to the toilet more frequently. Her friend's parents were woken up when she began vomiting, and when they noticed her looking pale and panting rapidly they brought her directly to hospital. Her friend's mother brought her to the Emergency Department, as her own parents were unable to be contacted at the time.

03:02–03:09 hours

Donna is assessed by the triage nurse and is moved into a cubicle inside the Emergency Department. Her friend's mother relays the night's events and the rapid onset of breathlessness, vomiting, abdominal pain and headache. Now she is becoming progressively drowsier. The nurse begins an assessment and, recognising the seriousness of the situation, calls for medical assistance early.

03:09 hours

You are writing up a patient's notes when a nurse calls you to see the new patient in cubicle 10. The nurse describes the history as you enter the cubicle to see Donna lying on the trolley. While listening to this quick history you are assessing her. Your first thought is that she looks unwell. She manages to confirm that she is diabetic, but that is the only direct history you can obtain.

A primary survey is performed: she is maintaining her airway and her breathing is rapid with deep, sighing breaths. You also notice her breath smells a bit like nail polish remover. You measure her respiratory rate at 35 breaths/min. Her pulse is weak and rapid with a rate of 130 bpm. Her capillary refill is slow (5 seconds), she has reduced skin turgor and you notice that her lips and oral mucosa appear dry—you suspect she is significantly dehydrated.

She is drowsy. Donna only opens her eyes in response to your voice—you assess her GCS as 13 (E3 V4 M6).

The nurse immediately applies high-flow oxygen via a non-rebreathing oxygen mask and applies monitoring: pulse oximeter, a blood pressure cuff and ECG monitoring.

Clinical question 1

(a) What is your immediate response? Describe how you will assess and manage Donna now.

(b) What is the diagnosis? Consider what could have precipitated this condition.

(c) What other information do you require at this stage? Make a list and justify your answers.

Physiology comment

There are two main types of diabetes: type 1 and type 2. Patients with type 1 diabetes can develop a condition known as DKA. Diabetic ketoacidosis is a metabolic state, caused by a diabetes-induced insulin deficit, which results in hyperglycaemia and plasma ketone bodies > 5 mmol/L. Insulin is an anabolic hormone and a deficit results in abnormal metabolism, which eventually leads to the mobilisation of lipids. As we will see later, frequent urination, rapid deep respirations (Kussmaul breathing), nausea and vomiting are all signs of a progressing insulin deficit and lead the treating physician to ask about any diabetic history.

A lack of insulin means that glucose cannot enter cells readily and the body has to rely on other food classes for energy production. Utilisation of lipids (and to a lesser extent proteins) instead of glucose as an energy substrate leads to fatty acids and their metabolites appearing in the blood at elevated levels. The metabolites are known as ketone bodies or ketoacids and consist of acetone and two organic acids (β-hydroxybutyric acid and acetoacetic acid). The acetone breath is caused by the elevated levels of these metabolites in the pulmonary capillary blood tainting the alveolar gas. The rapid, deep panting is caused by the body attempting to compensate for the metabolic acidosis caused by the accumulation of the ketoacids. Increasing the rate and depth of breathing and therefore blowing off carbon dioxide will partially compensate for the developing metabolic acidosis.

Patients with DKA typically have a fluid deficit of 3–5 litres upon admission. This level of volume loss is obviously significant and the likelihood of hypovolaemic shock developing should always be at the forefront of the treating physician's mind. Patients presenting with DKA also tend to be deficient in sodium and potassium, because of excessive losses in the urine. An osmotic diuresis in DKA is caused by an elevated glucose loading in the nephrons of the kidney The transport maximum of each nephron is overwhelmed by the unusually high glucose load and, instead of being fully reabsorbed by the end of the proximal tubule, glucose begins to enter the latter parts of the nephron. Glucose in the distal parts of the nephron tubule exerts an osmotic force, which causes the retention of water and associated ions in the collecting duct filtrate. This eventually leads to a pronounced osmotic diuresis and therefore frequent urination, one of the signs of diabetes.

Note: Serum values of electrolytes may be misleading in DKA, as water is lost along with electrolytes. Measured electrolyte concentrations may possibly be elevated even though there is an overall total body deficit. This is not because an increase in total body electrolyte has occurred, but because relatively more water than electrolyte has been lost. Care must be taken to always interpret electrolyte values along with an assessment of body fluid status.

03:14 hours

While the emergency nurse continues to apply monitoring, you do a quick fingertip-prick test for her BGL. Within 20 seconds the reading shows 'high'. The monitor provides the following information:

- SpO$_2$: 92%
- HR: 124 bpm
- BP: 90/55 mmHg

The diagnosis of DKA is clear. You recognise that Donna is shocked and that fluid resuscitation is necessary. You prepare to insert an intravenous cannula; however, she is significantly dehydrated and her veins have 'shut down', so venous access is difficult. Access is achieved after two attempts, and blood is collected from the cannula. The blood is sent to the pathology laboratory for urgent testing, and you request the following:

- blood glucose;
- urea/electrolytes/creatinine;
- full blood count;
- blood cultures.

03:22 hours

Estimating her weight at 40 kg, and referring to the guidelines from the Melbourne Royal Children's Hospital for fluid resuscitation in DKA, you immediately ask the nurse to give her 400 mL of 0.9% normal saline (40 kg × 10 mL/kg = 400 mL). You also write an infusion of 4 units per hour (0.1 U/kg/hour) of short-acting insulin to be administered intravenously.

A urine specimen is obtained and is tested.

03:30 hours

Wishing to better assess Donna's acid–base status, you take an arterial blood sample from her left radial artery. This can be a painful procedure—but tonight Donna is feeling so unwell she doesn't seem to notice.

The nurse returns with the dipstick urine result:

- ketones ++++
- leucocytes –
- nitrites –
- glucose ++++

Shortly afterwards the results of the ABG results become available (see Table 11.1).

Table 11.1 First arterial blood gas results

FIO$_2$	0.35
Blood gas values:	
pH	6.823
PaCO$_2$	11.5 mmHg
PaO$_2$	181 mmHg
BE	––
HCO$_3$$^-$	1.8 mmol/L
Electrolyte values:	
K$^+$	6.7 mmol/L
Na$^+$	123 mmol/L
Metabolite values:	
Glu	45 mmol/L
Lac	3.3 mmol/L

Clinical question 2

(a) Describe the ABG. It is indeed 'acidotic', but what else is there to note?

(b) Is the patient compensating appropriately?

(c) What does the ward urine test tell you about Donna's condition?

Clinical comment

Donna has a profound metabolic acidosis, and the low PaCO$_2$ of 11.5 indicates that she is trying very hard to compensate. However, with a pH < 7.0, this would be unlikely to occur. The elevated potassium should be noted: as will be discussed below, this can alter rapidly once therapy commences.

The ward urine test indicates ketonuria and glycosuria, which is diagnostic of DKA. Importantly there are no nitrites, suggesting that a urinary tract infection (a possible precipitant) is not present.

Physiology comment

The ABG data indicate severe metabolic acidosis and a raised potassium (normal 3.5–5.5 mmol/L) with a reduced sodium (normal = 136–146 mmol/L) level.

Sodium

Secondary to the acidosis, DKA patients may present with either hypo- or hyper-natraemia (*Note*: All patients will have a reduced total body sodium to some degree upon presentation). Hyponatraemia is more common and is resultant of a combination of:

- loss of sodium through osmotic diuresis;
- vomiting;
- hyperglycaemia-induced water shift from intracellular to extracellular compartments.

Elevated glucose can also interfere with the analysis procedure for plasma sodium, so plasma sodium levels need to be corrected to obtain a true value, by taking into account the coexisting plasma glucose concentration.

Potassium

Secondary to the ketone induced metabolic acidosis, several intracellular ions (such as potassium, phosphate and magnesium) will shift to the extracellular fluid in exchange for hydrogen ions across the cell membrane (in the case of potassium, leading to hyperkalaemia). This in itself may lead to an elevated renal loss through a higher filtered load at the glomeruli. The underlying hypokalaemic state usually becomes apparent only after insulin therapy converts the presenting hyperkalaemia to hypokalaemia.

03:40–05:00 hours

Although you will have to wait for the other blood tests (including blood cultures) to confirm the exact precipitant of the DKA, you can now begin further treatment to correct Donna's poor perfusion and consequently her metabolic acidosis. You estimate that she is more than 7% dehydrated. You order another bolus of 0.9% normal saline to improve her circulating volume and then begin calculating her maintenance fluid requirements, plus an intravenous insulin infusion to follow on from the bolus given earlier. The guidelines indicate that she should receive 162 mL of normal saline per hour to provide both replacement and maintenance fluid requirements.

By 04:00 hours she has received 800 mL of normal saline and seems to be improving clinically. You take a second arterial blood sample to assess progress (see Table 11.2).

Table 11.2 Second arterial blood gas results

FIO$_2$	0.35
Blood gas values:	
pH	7.13
PaCO$_2$	14.8 mmHg
PaO$_2$	225 mmHg
HCO$_3^-$	6.7 mmol/L
Electrolyte values:	
K$^+$	4.3 mmol/L
Na$^+$	122 mmol/L
Ca$^+$	1.31 mmol/L
Ca^{2+} (7.4)	0.91 mmol/L
Metabolite values:	
Glu	36 mmol/L
Lac	2.9 mmol/L

Clinical question 3

(a) Interpret this ABG and compare it to the previous result.
(b) Comment upon the K$^+$ result and discuss your clinical response.

Clinical comment

The acidosis is improving; however, as expected, the potassium is dropping. The potassium level must be monitored closely, as the blood level will drop precipitously once therapy begins and the potassium starts moving back into the cells. Potassium replacement should not be considered until the level falls below 5.5 mmol/L and the patient has passed urine—this has occurred, so intravenous potassium replacement should commence and close monitoring should continue.

Donna's clinical signs are improving: she is becoming more awake, her pulse rate is dropping, and her perfusion is improving. You contact the paediatric registrar to arrange admission to the ICU and to continue her treatment.

Epilogue

Later that day when the patient recovers you learn that she had not been taking her insulin for the last 36 hours because someone had told her it 'would make her fat'. Although the urine and blood cultures have yet to be finalised, you suspect that this misleading advice, in conjunction with the high sugar load she had consumed at the sleepover, was responsible for precipitating the DKA crisis.

Physiology comment

Overview of diabetic ketoacidosis

Management of an acute DKA episode links closely to the underlying physiological causes and an understanding is vital to appropriately treating a patient. Management is aimed at:

- restoring any intravascular volume loss that may lead to shock;
- control of blood glucose by using exogenous insulin;
- replacement of any potassium losses;
- correction of acid–base disturbance if severe;
- replacement of phosphate if significant.

An infusion of saline quickly re-expands the vascular space, correcting any life-threatening hypovolaemia. A treating physician should be aware that potassium levels may drop (leading to a life threatening hypokalaemia), secondary to any insulin therapy and therefore early potassium replacement may be warranted.

Correction of an underlying acid–base disturbance with bicarbonate therapy is controversial, as bicarbonate therapy *may* cause paradoxical central nervous system acidosis and rapid correction of acidosis caused by bicarbonate may result in hypokalaemia. Bicarbonate may be of use in selected patients with a pH < 6.9. Therapy is directed at correcting the underlying cause of the acidosis itself, rather than normalising the blood gas values.

Clinical comment

Donna presented with a severe episode of DKA. The diagnosis was been confirmed by:

- acidosis—low pH, low bicarbonate and elevated anion gap;
- hyperglycaemia—BGL > 15 mmol/L;
- clinical signs of altered conscious state; Kussmaul breathing, and hypovolaemic shock;
- ketonuria.

The diagnosis was easily made in this instance, thus allowing for early appropriate management. However, a significant proportion of undiagnosed diabetics present to hospital with ketoacidosis—that is, they are diagnosed with the condition only when they present critically unwell. It is therefore essential that Emergency Department staff consider DKA as a diagnosis in any young person who presents acutely unwell like this.

As in any situation, resuscitation is the essential first step; assessment and management of airway, breathing and circulation take priority. If the patient is unconscious and not protecting their airway, then intubation will need to be performed to provide definitive airway protection.

In this instance, fluid resuscitation followed well-established guidelines for the management of shock in children: a 10 mL/kg intravenous bolus of fluid was given. Once this is commenced there is time to calculate the fluid deficit and the ongoing fluid requirements. Clinicians must proceed with caution as cerebral oedema can result from incorrect fluid replacement, resulting in a high mortality.

Commencing insulin is an essential early step; and close attention must be paid to the potassium levels, which may drop precipitously once therapy starts and the acidosis begins to be corrected. Early consultation with senior specialist staff is important to guide therapy.

It is not enough to simply diagnose the condition and focus on the treatment of the ketoacidosis. While resuscitation and specific management of the DKA continue, attention should be paid to identifying and treating the precipitant. Common precipitants include poor compliance with insulin and diet, infection (viral or bacterial causes), some medication, and other intercurrent illnesses. Hence, the history and the examination should be directed towards identifying such conditions. In Donna's case, the history was obtained from the adult who brought her to hospital. Clinical examination and investigation may yield further clues. For example, a urine test may diagnose a urinary tract infection, or the presence of crackles on the chest combined with a fever would initiate a CXR, which would confirm the diagnosis of pneumonia. These conditions would obviously require specific therapy as treatment of the DKA itself continues.

It is also important that type 1 diabetics are treated appropriately in the early stages of any acute illness so that they do not ultimately progress into a ketoacidotic state when the risk of adverse outcomes is much higher.

Diabetic ketoacidosis, and diabetes in general, is a condition that affects multiple body systems and that requires a multidisciplinary approach to achieve optimal management. Early recognition of the condition and early referral to specialist multidisciplinary teams are the cornerstone of treatment.

References and further reading

1 Agus, M.S., Wolfsdorf, J.I. Diabetic ketoacidosis in children. Pediatr Clin North Am 2005 Aug; 52(4): 1147–63.
2 Charfen, M.A., Fernández-Frackelton, M. Diabetic ketoacidosis. Emerg Med Clin North Am 2005; 23(3): 609–28.
3 English, P., Williams, G. Hyperglycaemic crises and lactic acidosis in diabetes mellitus. Postgrad Med J 2004; 80: 253–61.
4 Glaser, N., Kuppermann, N. The evaluation and management of children with diabetic ketoacidosis in the emergency department. Pediatr Emerg Care 2004 July; 20(7): 477–81.
5 Guidelines from the Melbourne Royal Children's Hospital for fluid resuscitation in DKA. www.rch.org.au/clinicalguides
6 Koves, I.H., Neutze, J., Donath, S. et al. ESPE/LWPES consensus statement on diabetic ketoacidosis in children and adolescents. Archives of Disease in Childhood 2004; 89: 188–94. http://adc.bmjjournals.com/cgi/content/full/89/2/188?ijkey=19ff6d4260950d1dc5bb9f695475c2a6a9ffed51

Review

Level 1: Content knowledge

1 The osmotic diuresis in diabetic ketoacidosis (DKA) is caused by:
   A Increased filtered load of potassium
   B Increased filtered load of sodium
   C Increased filtered load of glucose
   D A lack of antidiuretic hormone

2 The acetone breath associated with DKA is caused by:
   A Haemoglobin breakdown
   B Lactic acid accumulation
   C Ketone bodies
   D Glucagon

3 Kussmaul breathing is a:
   A Slow shallow breathing pattern
   B Fast shallow breathing pattern
   C Slow deep breathing pattern
   D Fast deep breathing pattern

Level 2: Clinical applications

1 Which of the following findings would you *not* expect in a patient with severe DKA?
   A High BGL
   B High serum potassium
   C Normal anion gap
   D Rapid respirations
   E Clinically dehydrated

2 Which is the most common precipitant of DKA in children?
   A Urinary tract infection
   B Non-compliance with diet and therapy
   C Gastroenteritis producing vomiting and diarrhoea
   D Alcohol ingestion
   E Undiagnosed thyroid disease

3 Which of the following treatments is *not* recommended for the management of acute DKA in children?
   A Intravenous fluid resuscitation: 20 mL/kg bolus repeated until perfusion returns
   B Insulin infusion
   C Potassium replacement once serum potassium falls below 4.5 mmol/L

D Assessment of possible septic precipitants
E Frequent re-checking of blood glucose level

Level 3: Topics for further discussion

1 Discuss the appropriate mode of insulin replacement when treating DKA in your institution.

2 Discuss the multidisciplinary approach to managing adolescent patients with diabetes.

Case 12
Derek only occasionally used heroin …

Drug use appears in some unexpected places. Sometimes things go terribly wrong, as has occurred in this instance: a cascade of events leads to a life-threatening situation requiring rapid assessment and management. Multiple diagnostic and management dilemmas must be prioritised and addressed.

Timeline summary

12:05	Arrives at Emergency Department.
12:13	Triaged category 3: 'complains of painful legs'.
12:40	Seen by resident medical officer; commences assessment and initial management with intravenous fluid; first arterial blood sample taken.
12:50	Resident presents case to consultant
12:55	12-lead electrocardiogram (ECG) available; transferred to monitored bed.
13:00–13:15	Medication commenced; fluid resuscitation continues; arterial blood gas (ABG) results.
13:20	Central venous access obtained; indwelling catheter passed.
13:30	Pathology results available.
13:45	Improvement in condition; second ABG taken.
14:10	Reviewed by plastic surgery and intensive care teams.

Learning objectives

Physiological

- Define rhabdomyolysis and how it relates to this case.
- Describe the difference between internal and external potassium balance and how rhabdomyolysis can influence potassium distribution in the body.
- Understand how hyperkalaemia can alter cardiac conduction.
- Outline the physiological basis of using insulin for treating hyperkalaemia.
- Understand how rhabdomyolysis can lead to kidney failure.

Clinical

- Recognise the features of life-threatening electrolyte disturbances on an ECG.
- Be able to prioritise clinical problems when confronted with a patient with multiple medical conditions.
- Know the causes of hyperkalaemia and describe how it is managed in an emergency situation.

Context

Derek only occasionally used heroin. He would have a shot of the illegal opiate every fortnight or so, in the same way someone might have a couple of beers at the local hotel. He'd been doing it for a few years now and was the perfect image of a young man doing good things with his life: he had a beautiful girlfriend, he was well regarded in his chosen career, and he lived in an apartment close to town. His future was promising and, at 26 years of age, Derek felt as if life was perfect.

Last Friday night was similar to many he'd had previously—he went to a friend's place and after a couple of hours retreated to a bedroom and injected $50 worth of heroin. He drifted off into a heroin-induced coma on the floor where he sat.

His friends found him late the next morning. They were used to him passing out, so did not pay too much attention to the fact he had been unconscious for nearly 12 hours. He was breathing rapidly, and appeared to be slowly coming out of his stupor. Eventually he awoke—but he complained that he couldn't move his legs. His friends tried to help him, but his legs were markedly swollen and he couldn't feel them. Something wasn't right—so they carried him into a car and drove him to the local Emergency Department.

169

12:13 hours

Derek has been triaged 'category 3—c/o painful legs' upon his arrival. His friends have brought him in on a wheelchair appropriated from the front of the Emergency Department. He has complained of difficulty walking, but he doesn't want to publicise what had really happened. He is directed to a cubicle in the department, and after 10 minutes a nurse recorded his observations. Again, he has kept his heroin use a secret—he doesn't want it to become common knowledge. This is a small town, and it is quite likely he will meet up with someone he knows. Just under 30 minutes after his arrival, he is seen by a resident medical officer.

12:40 hours

The resident looks at Derek (who has drifted off to sleep again) and looks at the vital signs as recorded by the nurse:

- PR: 110 bpm
- BP: 80/50 mmHg
- RR: 28 breaths/min
- temperature: 37.4°C

She goes to rouse Derek—who only responds with a groan. A harder shake brings him fully awake.

Doctor: 'Hi Derek – I'm the doctor … what's brought you here?'

Derek: 'Huh? Oh, I feel sick …'

Doctor: 'Are you OK, Derek? What's going on? You told the nurses you can't walk.'

Derek: 'Can you keep a secret?' The doctor nodded. 'I took some heroin last night and it was a bit much for me … I slept bent on my legs the whole night and now I can't walk …'

The resident looks more closely at Derek. He has dry cracked lips and a coated tongue, his breathing is shallow and rapid, and his legs are swollen and tense. She goes to feel pulses on his feet but can feel nothing.

Clinical question 1

(a) What is your initial impression of Derek and his condition?

(b) What are the possibilities?

(c) How will you proceed from here?

The resident thinks quickly but carefully. Whatever the cause of his condition, he looks sick. She commences some basic interventions while she thinks about her next move. She places a non-rebreathing oxygen mask at 15 L/min, and goes to find the cannulation trolley. She places a wide bore intravenous line into his right arm and commences a normal saline infusion; she takes a series of blood tests; and she takes an arterial blood sample for analysis. She hasn't been working in the Emergency Department for very long, but she is aware of her responsibilities and the need to discuss patients early with a consultant.

Clinical question 2

(a) What blood tests would you request?
(b) What would you expect to see on the ABG results?
(c) How would you present this case to the consultant?

Clinical comment

It is important to be able to recognise the seriously ill patient and to react appropriately and call for senior assistance early. Junior staff working in Emergency Departments are briefed to call for help in emergencies, regardless of how much has been determined about the cause of the patient's condition. As has been demonstrated in the previous cases, management can be started regardless of the final diagnosis; this patient is obviously displaying the clinical signs of poor tissue perfusion and is in the early stages of shock.

Initial actions should be based around the assessment and management of the patient's airway, breathing and circulation. He is alert and able to talk, indicating a patent airway. He is tachypnoeic, so oxygen would be a useful intervention until further information is acquired. Given his shocked state it may actually be that the tachypnoea represents respiratory compensation for a significant metabolic acidosis. The presence of tachycardia, hypotension and poor perfusion suggests that fluid resuscitation should be commenced once intravenous access has been obtained.

The shock could be due to a number of causes, but the swollen lower limbs should alert the clinician to compartment syndrome; lower limb thrombus with subsequent pulmonary embolism is also a possibility.

The cause should become apparent from taking a directed history from the patient.

Bloods collected should be sent to pathology and investigations requested which test the clinical hypotheses. The main pathology tests of interest would be urea and electrolytes (assessing potassium and renal function), creatine kinase and calcium (assessing for rhabdomyolysis), and a baseline full blood count and coagulation profile.

12:50 hours

The resident collects the bloods and proceeds to the doctor's station. As she labels the bloods and prepares to send them off to the pathology department, she presents Derek's story to the consultant emergency physician:

'Derek's quite unwell and I need your input and assistance. He's been unconscious overnight and has slept on his bent legs … he's almost in shock, he looks terribly dehydrated, and I think he's acidotic. His legs are tight and there's almost no perfusion in his lower legs. I've taken bloods for FBC, U & E's, LFT's, CK and coagulation profile. I've also started some normal saline intravenously. I'm quite worried about him.'

The consultant looked concerned. 'Sounds like you've got to the bottom of it pretty quickly and you're doing everything properly. Can you tie it all together into a single diagnosis?'

The resident thought for a moment. 'I'd be worried about a compartment syndrome in his lower legs … and that could lead to rhabdomyolysis …'

'Good,' said the consultant. 'What is his potassium concentration?'

Physiology comment

Rhabdomyolysis is an acute disease characterised by the destruction of skeletal muscle. Muscle damage can occur due to arterial occlusion (inadequate perfusion), direct compression leading to increased compartment pressure (disruption of cell membrane) or direct mechanical disruption of the cell. The result of the cell damage is the release of a range of substances including lactic acid, potassium, myoglobin, uric acid, phosphate, histamine, leukotrienes and markers such as creatine kinase. The lack of perfusion while Derek was unconscious led to localised muscle damage in his legs. The resultant swelling and impaired distal perfusion has led to rhabdomyolysis.

12:55 hours

Before the resident can answer, the nurse arrives with the 12-lead ECG and shows it to the consultant (see Fig. 12.1).

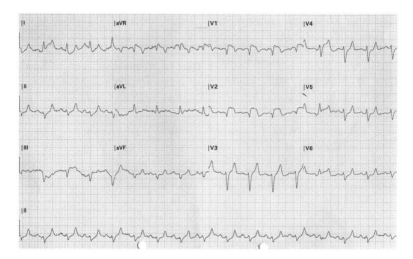

Figure 12.1 ECG

Clinical question 3

(a) Interpret the ECG.
(b) What do you think his K⁺ could be?
(c) What are the immediate management priorities?
(d) What therapy would you commence?

The consultant interpreted the ECG:

'Peaked T-waves, widened QRS and a prolonged QT interval. He must have potassium of at least 8 mmol/L. We'd better start treating him urgently.'

The patient is rapidly moved to a monitored bed in the high dependency area of the department, where he can be monitored constantly and there is a higher nurse-to-patient ratio.

13:00 hours

The consultant writes up medication to deal with Derek's life-threatening hyperkalaemia. The drugs in Table 12.1 are prescribed for immediate administration.

Table 12.1 Medication administration

Once-only medications

Date	Medication	Dose	Route	Date to be given	Time to be given	Signed	Given by
23/5	Calcium gluconate	1 g	IV	23/5/05	1255	GC	
23/5	Salbutamol	5 mg	Nebulised	23/5/05	1255	GC	
23/5	8.4% NaHCO$_3$	50 mL	IV	23/5/05	1255	GC	
23/5	50% Dextrose	25 mL	IV	23/5/05	1255	GC	
23/5	Insulin (Actrapid)	10 U	IV	23/5/05	1255	GC	

The nurse returns with the ABG taken a few minutes previously (see Table 12.2).

Table 12.2 First arterial blood gas results

FIO$_2$	0.35
Blood gas values:	
pH	7.075
PaCO$_2$	15.0 mmHg
PaO$_2$	134 mmHg
BE	−24.5 mmol/L
HCO$_3^-$	4.2 mmol/L
Oximetry values:	
Hb	179 g/L
SaO$_2$	97.0%
Electrolyte values:	
K$^+$	7.8 mmol/L
Na$^+$	131 mmol/L
Ca^{2+}	0.91 mmol/L
Ca^{2+} (7.4)	0.75 mmol/L
Metabolite values:	
Glu	5.8 mmol/L
Lac	5.6 mmol/L

Clinical question 4

Interpret the ABG results.

Clinical comment

This patient appears to have compartment syndrome of his lower limbs as a result of hours of pressure and inactivity. The muscle has swollen and necrosed, impeding distal circulation. There has been a massive release of potassium into the circulation; this has been unable to be excreted due to renal dysfunction, thereby amplifying the condition.

The ECG is used as both a diagnostic and a prognostic tool for hyperkalaemia. Features of hyperkalaemia on ECG include peaked T waves, widened QRS and a prolonged QT interval. As the potassium rises the ECG adopts a 'sinusoidal' shape as the QRS complex and T waves alter. The hyperkalaemia is the most important clinical condition present and must be dealt with urgently.

A metabolic acidosis would be expected on the ABG. However, the ABG has an immediately practical component in that it often allows for a rapid potassium result to be obtained, thus confirming one of the key diagnoses. This ABG reveals a lactic metabolic acidosis, an attempt to compensate by hyperventilation, and elevated haemoglobin (indicating haemoconcentration from dehydration).

Physiology comment

Potassium distribution

Approximately 98% of potassium is located within the cells due to active transport of potassium into cells across the cell membrane. Movement of potassium across the cell membrane is, to some extent, under physiological control and the resultant proportion of intracellular to extracellular potassium is termed the 'internal balance' or the 'internal distribution'. Extracellular plasma concentration is therefore determined by a combination of external balance (input versus output primarily regulated by the renal system) and internal balance. Cell damage as in the case of rhabdomyolysis leads to a massive increase in the extracellular potassium concentration as intracellular potassium from damaged cells leaks out into the extracellular compartment. The major factors that regulate internal balance are adrenaline and insulin and in cases of extensive cell damage increased adrenaline levels offset the hyperkalaemia to some degree by increasing potassium uptake by non-damaged cells.

Hyperkalaemia and cardiac conduction

The ratio of intracellular to extracellular potassium ion concentration is a major determinant of the resting membrane potential (RMP) of muscle cells. Changes in this internal potassium balance therefore caused altered function of smooth, skeletal and in particular cardiac muscle. Abnormal plasma concentrations of potassium (that is, hypo- and hyperkalaemia) can produce marked changes to cardiac conduction and therefore the ECG. Hyperkalaemia produces ECG changes associated with both depolarisation and repolarisation. Initially, narrowing and peaking of the T waves is often seen; the PR interval then becomes prolonged and in severe hyperkalaemia widened QRS complexes are seen. These changes in the ECG are related to the alteration in extracellular to intracellular potassium ratio. The hyperkalaemia decreases the duration of cardiac action potentials and decreases conduction velocity through cells in the heart. In addition the increase in extracellular potassium effectively decreases the RMP of cardiac cells; in extreme cases the RMP can exceed the cell's threshold potential and the cell cannot repolarise and will not respond to stimulation and contract.

The consultant introduces himself to the patient. 'Hi Derek, I'm one of the senior doctors here. How are you feeling?'

Derek looks at the doctor miserably. 'I feel really sick. What's going on?'

The consultant looks him in the eyes. 'I'm worried that you've got muscle damage from where you were lying on your legs overnight. That muscle has broken down and has damaged your kidneys. Your potassium is quite high, and I'm also worried that your legs are quite swollen and are cutting off the blood supply to your feet.'

He looks at Derek's legs, which are swollen and pale. He turns to the resident. 'I think we should ask the plastic surgeons to come and have a look—we need to do urgent fasciotomies.'

Clinical question 5

(a) Formulate a problem list for Derek as you see it now. Prioritise your tasks, and think about how you will manage each of them in a coordinated and integrated fashion.

(b) Discuss the rationale for the management of hyperkalaemia.

(c) What are the complications of hyperkalaemia?

Clinical comment

Derek is seriously ill. His problem list would look like this:

- hyperkalaemia;
- rhabdomyolysis;
- compartment syndrome in both legs;
- acute renal failure.

The lack of perfusion in Derek's leg while he was unconscious led to localised muscle damage in his legs, which in turn has caused marked swelling and impaired distal perfusion. The breakdown of muscle has caused intracellular potassium to be released (amongst other metabolites, such as creatinine kinase), and this in turn has caused acute renal failure.

The immediate management would be focused on:

- rapidly reducing the serum potassium and preventing the serious complications of ventricular fibrillation and death;
- aggressive intravenous fluid therapy to restore systemic perfusion;
- urgent surgical consultation to perform fasciotomies, so that the distal blood flow can be restored and the limbs can be saved;
- urgent intensive care consultation so that dialysis can be arranged.

Note that the complete blood results are not required prior to initiating management—in an emergency, assessment and management occur in parallel. The diagnosis of hyperkalaemia was suspected from the clinical presentation and confirmed by the ECG changes—therapy started before the level was actually available.

13:20 hours

The medications to immediately reduce Derek's potassium level have been given, and an insulin/dextrose infusion is started. Central venous access is obtained by placing a triple-lumen subclavian central line, and aggressive fluid management is initiated (see Table 12.3).

Table 12.3 Fluid orders table

Date	Fluid	Additives	Volume	Rate	Medical officer	Commenced
23/5/05	N/S	Nil	1 litre	STAT	GC	
23/5/05	N/S	Nil	1 litre	STAT	GC	
23/5/05	N/S	Nil	1 litre	STAT	GC	

Physiology comment

Physiological basis of using insulin and dextrose for treating hyperkalaemia

Management is aimed at antagonising the cardio-toxic effect of potassium, shifting potassium into cells and enhancing potassium excretion. Insulin, catecholamines, aldosterone and alkalosis all stimulate potassium uptake by cells, therefore altering the internal balance of potassium. Insulin is commonly used to treat hyperkalaemia; the mechanism by which insulin (administered with glucose to prevent hypoglycaemia) shifts potassium into cells is not fully understood, but it is thought to be related to stimulation of the Na-K-ATPase.

An indwelling catheter is inserted, but only a trickle of brownish-coloured urine appears. The urine is tested and is strongly positive for blood.

13:30 hours

The haematology and biochemistry results become available (see Table 12.4).

Table 12.4 Haematology and biochemistry results

Haematology values:	
Hb	195 High
RCC	6.31 High
Hct	58 High
WCC	28.8 High Neut
	23.9 High Left shift
Plat	216
Coagulation profile:	
INR	1.2 High
Fib	7.85 High
D-Dim	Positive
Electrolyte values:	
K$^+$	7.5 High
Na$^+$	130 Low
Cl$^-$	99
HCO$_3^-$	21 Low
Urea	22.5 High
Creat	485 High

Clinical question 6

(a) Interpret and comment upon the blood results.
(b) Are they what you expected?

Clinical comment

The blood results are consistent with the clinical condition described:

- The elevated haemoglobin suggests significant haemoconcentration, caused by dehydration.
- A raised white cell count indicates an acute inflammatory response.
- The elevated urea and creatinine in combination with a low bicarbonate is indicative of acute renal failure.
- An elevated creatinine kinase, released by the breakdown of skeletal muscle, is diagnostic of rhabdomyolysis.
- The elevated K$^+$ is indeed confirmed.

Physiology comment

Rhabdomyolysis and kidney failure

Acute renal failure occurs when there is a rapid drop in glomerular filtration rate and therefore renal function. In rhabdomyolysis, acute renal failure can often develop (in 10–15% of cases) as a result of increased plasma haemoglobin and myoglobin levels and therefore the renal filtered load of these proteins. There are a number of mechanisms by which kidney damage can occur either directly or indirectly. The toxicity of haemoglobin and myoglobin is increased by low tubular flows and concentrated tubular fluid secondary to volume depletion.

13:45 hours

Derek has received aggressive fluid resuscitation, and his ECG has improved, suggesting that the medication has been successful in moving the potassium back into the cells. A repeat arterial blood sample is taken (see Table 12.5).

Table 12.5 Third arterial blood gas results

O_2 via mask at 6 L/min	>0.21
Blood gas values:	
pH	7.12
$PaCO_2$	25 mmHg
PaO_2	143 mmHg
BE	−19.6 mmol/L
HCO_3^-	6.4 mmol/L
Electrolyte values:	
K^+	5.8 mmol/L
Na^+	130 mmol/L
Ca^+	0.90 mmol/L
Metabolite values:	
Glu	11.6 mmol/L
Lac	4.9 mmol/L

14:10 hours

The plastic surgeon has seen the patient in the Emergency Department, and has made arrangements to perform fasciotomies once his potassium is corrected and he is safe for a general anaesthetic. Knowing that the reduction in potassium is just a temporary measure, the intensive care specialists are preparing to commence dialysis as soon as a bed is available in the intensive care unit.

Epilogue

Derek had a difficult course in hospital: the fasciotomies were unable to restore perfusion to his lower limbs. Examination under a general anaesthetic revealed significant muscle necrosis. He went to the operating theatre several times in attempts to save his legs, but this was ultimately unsuccessful. He eventually had bilateral above-knee amputations.

He was in intensive care for approximately 6 weeks, during which time he was on renal dialysis. His kidneys eventually recovered to the point that dialysis could be stopped. He was discharged to the ward and then referred to orthotic and rehabilitation specialists for fitting prosthetic legs and to learn how to walk again.

Clinical comment

This patient presented with multiple problems, interrelated but each requiring urgent, specific, and coordinated management. He presented in a shocked state, and looked unwell. The resident recognised this, sought assistance from senior colleagues, and started appropriate basic resuscitation treatment: oxygen administration, intravenous access and intravenous fluid therapy. The serious nature of the condition was suggested by the history and physical examination, and the ECG followed by the blood gas confirmed the diagnosis. In this circumstance, as has happened in most other cases described in this book, assessment and management have occurred in parallel. The practice of emergency medicine is such that treatment often has to begin before all information is available.

Hyperkalaemia

This patient has dangerously high potassium, as evidenced by the significant ECG changes. Hyperkalaemia broadly results from an excess production of potassium or a reduction in the renal clearance of potassium, or, as has happened in this instance, a potent combination of the two. Skeletal muscle necrosis has released large amounts of potassium into the circulation, and the combination of dehydration and circulating myoglobins contributing to acute renal failure has produced a hyperkalaemic state. Initial therapy is directed towards preventing cardiac arrhythmias and moving the potassium back into the cells. Calcium gluconate must be administered first, not because of any effect on the potassium level, but for its cardiac-stabilising properties so that dangerous cardiac rhythms may be prevented. There is good evidence that the combination of salbutamol together with insulin and dextrose is effective in rapidly decreasing the serum potassium level. However, pharmacological therapy only provides temporary respite. If there is an increased load of potassium in the body and the kidneys are unable to clear it, then the potassium must be removed by another means: dialysis.

Rhabdomyolysis and compartment syndrome

Skeletal muscle can be damaged by a number of different mechanisms, but Derek's circumstance is essentially similar to the crush injuries sustained by people trapped under rubble and heavy weights. The necrosed muscle releases myoglobin, which causes direct damage to renal glomeruli. The affected muscle compartments swell as a result of reduced perfusion, increasing intra-compartment pressure, thus further reducing distal perfusion and causing even more muscle necrosis. A metabolic acidosis results as toxic metabolites accumulate. This is reflected in the ABG. Early fasciotomies to restore blood flow and debridement of necrosed tissue are the principles of surgical therapy. A surgical opinion must be sought urgently if this condition is suspected. If the diagnosis is in doubt the intra-compartmental pressure may be measured, with a pressure greater than 35 mmHg suggestive of compartment syndrome.

The diagnosis of rhabdomyolysis is confirmed by an elevated creatinine kinase and the presence of myoglobins in the urine. However, rhabdomy- olysis and compartment syndrome are essentially clinical diagnoses.

Renal failure

As mentioned above, the combination of hypovolaemia, acidosis and myoglobin release leads to acute renal failure. Early aggressive restoration of perfusion with intravenous fluid treatment, coupled with attempts to alkalinise the urine may reduce the impact of these insults.

Summary

Rhabdomyolysis is a medical emergency, and is associated with significant morbidity and mortality. The doctor working in the Emergency Depart- ment must be aware of potential complications arising from such a condition, and be prepared to look for the expected sequelae.

References and further reading

1 Bontempo, L. Rhabdomyolysis. Chapter 121, pp. 1762–70. In Marx, J.A. (ed.), *Rosen's Emergency Medicine: Concepts and Clinical Practice.* 5th edn. St Louis, Mosby, 2002.
2 Gonzalez, D. Crush syndrome. Crit Care Med 2005; 33[Suppl.]: S34–41.
3 Mahoney, B.A., Smith, W.A.D., Lo, D.S., Tsoi, K., Tonelli, M., Clase, C.M. Emergency interventions for hyperkalaemia. The Cochrane Database of Systematic Reviews 2005; Issue 2. Art. No.: CD003235.pub2.
4 Singh, D., Chander, V., Chopra, K. Rhabdomyolysis. Methods Find Exp Clin Pharmacol 2005; 27(1): 39–48.

Review

Level 1: Content knowledge

1 Rhabdomyolysis is an acute disease characterised by:
   A The destruction of heart muscle
   B The destruction of smooth muscle
   C The destruction of skeletal muscle
   D Unaltered electrolyte values

2 In rhabdomyolysis, acute renal failure can develop as a result of:
   A Increased filtered load of haemoglobin and myoglobin
   B Hypovolaemic shock
   C Immune damage to the filtration barrier
   D Stenosis of the renal artery

3 The following factors stimulate potassium cellular uptake:
   A Insulin, catecholamines, aldosterone and acidosis
   B Insulin, glucagon, aldosterone and alkalosis
   C Insulin, glucagon, aldosterone and acidosis
   D Insulin, catecholamines, aldosterone and alkalosis

Level 2: Clinical applications

1 Which of the following is the most appropriate first therapy for a patient with ECG changes due to hyperkalaemia?
   A 5 mg nebulised salbutamol
   B 1 g of intravenous calcium gluconate
   C 30 g of oral resonium resin
   D 50 mL of intravenous 8.4% sodium bicarbonate
   E 100 µg of intravenous salbutamol

2 After giving the above medication, indicate which of the following interventions are the most appropriate to commence and in what order:
   A Nebulised salbutamol, intravenous dextrose
   B Intravenous bicarbonate
   C 30 g of oral resonium resin
   D Urgent dialysis
   E Intravenous salbutamol and intravenous frusemide

3 Which of the following results would *not* be expected in a patient with rhabdomyolysis?
   A Prolonged QT interval on ECG
   B Hypocalcaemia
   C Metabolic acidosis

D Metabolic alkalosis

E Myoglobinuria

Level 3: Topics for further discussion

1 The acute identification and management of electrolyte disturbances is essential in the practice of emergency medicine. Discuss the different abnormalities that can occur and be familiar with their emergency management.

2 Discuss the team approach to managing a patient with multiple life-threatening problems.

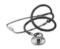

Integrated questions

1 Match the following clinical conditions and the most appropriate pathophysiological classification of shock:

  A A young female injures her chest in a fall and is tachycardic and breathless; her trachea is deviated to the left and she has reduced breath sounds on the right.

  B A female is in a motor vehicle crash, has extensive bruising on the left side of her body, complains of left upper quadrant pain and is hypotensive.

  C A person is stabbed in the left fifth intercostal space in the mid-clavicular line and is hypotensive and tachycardic.

  D An elderly male collapses after complaining of chest pain; his ECG reveals ST segment elevation in leads II, III and aVF.

  E A child is stung by a jack jumper ant and collapses shortly after-wards with a swollen face and a widespread erythematous rash.

  F A young female suffers burns to 50% of her body in a petrol explosion.

  G An elderly male on warfarin passes black tarry stools and is pale and sweaty.

  H A patient receives a spinal anaesthetic for an elective surgical procedure and is hypotensive.

  I An elderly male collapses 2 weeks after a total hip replacement; he is breathless, tachycardic and has a swollen left leg.

  J A 2-year-old boy is pale and lethargic after 2 days of watery diarrhoea and vomiting.

  K A young male becomes confused and drowsy. He is rushed to hospital and is found to have a widespread purpuric rash and a temperature of 38.3°C.

    (i) Hypovolaemic shock

    (ii) Cardiogenic shock

    (iii) Obstructive shock

    (iv) Distributive shock

2 In which of the following clinical conditions is analysis of blood gas *least* likely to assist with diagnosis and management?

A An elderly male with exacerbation of emphysema

B A young child with a moderate wheeze relieved by salbutamol

C An unconscious male pulled from a house fire

D An elderly woman with severe shortness of breath and left upper lobe consolidation on chest radiography

E A female with type 1 diabetes presenting with polyuria, polydipsia and hyperventilation

3 Match the clinical condition and the most useful initial diagnostic modality employed to assess it:

A A young female presents with polydipsia and polyuria.

B A 45-year-old male presents with central crushing chest pain radiating down his left arm.

C A 17-year-old male presents with a sudden onset of sharp, left-sided chest pain, is found to have reduced breath sounds and is hyper-resonant to percussion over his left upper chest.

D A 23-year-old male is found semi-conscious inside his motor vehicle, which is still running.

E An 18-year-old male presents with an exacerbation of asthma relieved by his salbutamol. He can talk in sentences and has been admitted to hospital previously.

   (i) Chest radiography

   (ii) Troponin

  (iii) D-dimer

   (iv) Blood glucose level

    (v) 12-lead ECG

   (vi) Dip-stick urine

  (vii) Spirometry

 (viii) Arterial blood gas with carboxy-haemoglobin analysis

4 Match the clinical condition described with the most likely ECG finding:

A A 43-year-old male complains of palpitations for the last 6 hours.

B A 17-year-old female presents with breathlessness and clinically has pneumonia.

C A 58-year-old female complains of heavy chest pain radiating to her jaw for the last 45 minutes and is sweaty and breathless.

D An 83-year-old male presents with acute renal failure secondary to a bowel obstruction.

E A 24-year-old male takes an overdose of 90 carbamazepine tablets and has a Glasgow coma score of 14.

F A 45-year-old male complained of 10 minutes of central chest pain 2 hours ago, but has had no pain since.

   (i) Normal ECG

   (ii) An irregular tracing with no P waves

   (iii) Sinus rhythm with peaked T waves

   (iv) Sinus rhythm with ST segment elevation in leads V_{2-5}

   (v) Ventricular tachycardia

   (vi) Sinus tachycardia with no other abnormalities

   (vii) Sinus tachycardia with a widened QRS and prolonged Q_T interval

   (viii) Sinus bradycardia

5 Match the diagnosis with the most appropriate definitive therapy:

  A Acute ST elevation myocardial infarction with hypoperfusion

  B Hyperkalaemia secondary to rhabdomyolysis

  C Cardiac arrest secondary to suspected pulmonary embolism

  D Acute pulmonary oedema with respiratory distress

  E Persistent hypotension secondary to liver injury in a motor vehicle crash

   (i) CPAP and GTN infusion

   (ii) Percutaneous coronary intervention (PCI) with angioplasty

   (iii) Renal dialysis after emergency management initiated

   (iv) Urgent transfer to operating theatre for laparotomy

   (v) Thrombolytic therapy

6 Match the following ABG results with the clinical condition that would most likely produce them:

No.	FIO_2	pH (7.35–7.45)	PCO_2 (35–45 mmHg)	PO_2 (mmHg)	HCO_3 (mmol/L)	Carboxy-haemoglobin (%)	K^+
(i)	0.28	7.04	84	62	29	5.6	3.9
(ii)	0.35	7.44	16	45	22	1.7	4.4
(iii)	0.21	7.16	17	102	5	1.1	3.9
(iv)	0.50	7.26	48	157	19	2.3	3.8
(v)	0.60	7.37	36	298	22	24.9	4.3
(vi)	1.00	6.89	33	67	1.2	3.4	8.7

  A A 76-year-old male is acutely breathless; the diagnosis of acute pulmonary oedema is made.

  B A 67-year-old female with emphysema is increasingly breathless and is brought to the hospital semi-conscious after 2 days of cough and increasing wheeze.

C A young female is diagnosed with severe community acquired pneumonia.

D A middle-aged male is found unconscious in his motor vehicle.

E A 15-year-old boy is brought to the Emergency Department after 2 days of polyuria and thirst.

F A patient has a cardiac arrest after being trapped by his lower legs in a motor vehicle crash for several hours, and resuscitation is taking place.

Answers

Case 1 review

Level 1: Content knowledge

1 D Total peripheral resistance increases due to the greater sympathetic outflow mediated via the baroreceptors.

2 A Note that B and C represent the values you would expect in cardiogenic and distributive shock, respectively.

3 D The shift from compensation to decompensation is determined by two variables: magnitude and duration of blood loss. An increase in either leads to greater initial peripheral vasoconstriction and ischaemic damage.

Level 2: Clinical applications

1 D All of the others are recognised as being at high risk of life-threatening injuries.

2 The purpose of this question is to alert emergency doctors of possible injuries based upon trauma patterns prior to the arrival of the patient.

  A (ii)
  B (v)
  C (iii)
  D (i)
  E (iv)

3 D This sequence most closely follows the ABCDE of the primary survey.

Level 3: Topics for further discussion

1 Trauma is a disease that requires an effective multidisciplinary approach in order to optimise care and outcomes. This care starts in the pre-hospital arena and a seamless transition through the system is desirable. Doctors should study trauma systems carefully to appreciate the factors that can influence patient care. Be aware of the different

epidemiology of trauma: blunt injury due to road crashes is the dominant pattern in rural Australia, whereas penetrating trauma from firearms or stabbings is more common in inner-city services. This will have an impact on hospital planning and resource allocation. The use of simulation centres allows for various scenarios to be practised in teams without the risk of adverse patient outcomes, and review and reflection can further improve performance.

2   Different intravenous fluids are used by different clinicians in different parts of the world at different times of the treatment process. However, the basic goal is similar: to restore perfusion while definitive care is being organised. In most instances operative therapy is not required, thus challenging the concept that 'trauma is a surgical disease'. In Australia, crystalloid fluids are used, with 0.9% normal saline being the preferred intravenous fluid of many clinicians. Colloids are rarely used in acute trauma management.

Case 2 review

Level 1: Content knowledge

1   B   In cardiac failure increased circulating volume can lead to a decrease in cardiac output due to damage to the heart tissue itself.

2   D   Options A, B and C are all causes of shortness of breath.

3   A   In aortic stenosis, a pressure gradient develops across the damaged valve as the left ventricle is forced to generate an increased pressure to overcome the stenosed opening.

Level 2: Clinical applications

1   B   ACE inhibitors improve mortality in patients with CCF and should be used routinely.

2   E   All of the other symptoms are suggestive of cardiac failure; haemoptysis should raise the possibility of infection or malignancy.

3   E   The other investigations should be used first to confirm diagnosis and to identify possible precipitants. Spirometry may have a role to assess alternative diagnoses.

4   **A**   (iv)
    B   (iii)
    C   (i)
    D   (ii)
    E   (vi)
    F   (v)

Level 3: Topics for further discussion

1 Decompensated cardiac failure can have adverse outcomes, so prevention of deterioration is an essential component of the chronic care of patients. Optimising medication and recognising precipitants is an essential part of optimally managing patients with cardiac failure.

2 The management of heart failure has advanced significantly in recent years, and it is essential that medical practitioners keep up to date with the latest advances and evidence. The Cochrane Library is a useful source of clinical information. Different classes of drugs such as angiotensin converting enzyme inhibitors, diuretics and beta-blockers are available to improve patient quality of life.

Case 3 review

Level 1: Content knowledge

1 D   As clotting is favoured by the conditions found in the leg and pelvic veins most emboli originate from these sites.

2 E

3 B   A normal PaO_2 is typically to be 5 to 15 mmHg below the alveolar value. Thus the $P(A-a)O_2$ is typically 5–15 mmHg. Pulmonary oedema can cause the $P(A-a)O_2$ to widen, indicating impaired gas exchange.

Level 2: Clinical applications

1 D   Although there may sometimes be features of right heart strain, sinus tachycardia is the most common ECG finding.

2 E   All are risk factors. The presence of risk factors can assist with calculating the clinical likelihood of embolic disease and can assist in the interpretation of investigations.

3 B   This patient is at high risk of a pulmonary thromboembolism, and the clinical value of this investigation declines in this circumstance. In other words, a negative D-dimer would not rule out the disease. A chest X-ray is performed to exclude other causes such as pneumonia or pneumothorax, as is the 12-lead ECG.

Level 3: Topics for further discussion

1 Computerised tomography is becoming increasingly used for the diagnosis of pulmonary embolism, and indications and interpretation data are constantly being updated. Pulmonary angiography is rarely used now, and ventilation/perfusion scanning is available only in

certain centres. Some authors advocate a combination of clinical risk factors and D-dimers to assign risk, but caution must be exercised when applying such rules to undifferentiated emergency patients.

2 Anticoagulation has been the standard therapy for pulmonary embolism for many years, but thrombolysis is becoming increasingly used for sub-massive emboli. This needs to be discussed carefully and the evidence assessed before it becomes widespread practice.

Case 4 review

Level 1: Content knowledge

1 C

2 C The underlying hypoxaemia seen in pneumonia is caused by V/Q mismatching (decreased alveolar ventilation is due to consolidation of acini) and diffusion impairment (caused by damage to the alveolar/capillary membrane).

3 B Hyperventilation will lead to a low $PaCO_2$ as ventilation regulates the amount of CO_2 blown off from the lungs. Hypercapnia may occur later in pneumonia if the patient becomes too exhausted to ventilate adequately.

Level 2: Clinical applications

1 C *Streptococcus pneumoniae* or 'pneumococcus' remains the most common cause of community-acquired pneumonia.

2 **A** (ii)
  B (v)
  C (i)
  D (iv)
  E (iii)

Note: It is recommended that readers check local protocols and sensitivities before using the above medications in a clinical setting.

3 A Note that B and E suggest cardiac failure; C suggests emphysema; and D suggests *Staphylococcus* infection.

Level 3: Topics for further discussion

1 The Pneumonia Severity Index (PSI—see the reference Johnson et al. 2002 in Case 4) is a helpful guide that can assist clinicians in applying an evidence-based risk stratification system when treating patients with CAP. It allows for evidence-based drug therapy to be used, thus

counteracting the growing problem of antibiotic resistance, and assists in the allocation of increasingly scarce health resources.

2 Pathology and public health staff can inform clinicians of disease epidemiology and antimicrobial resistance patterns in local regions and can therefore play a central role in managing infectious disease effectively.

Case 5 review

Level 1: Content knowledge

1 A

2 D The haemoglobin saturation gives information about the percentage of the available haem-binding sites that have been occupied.

3 A When a molecule of oxygen binds with haem a conformational change occurs (allosteric effect), increasing the affinity of the next binding site for oxygen.

Level 2: Clinical applications

1 **A** (iii)
   B (vi)
   C (v)
   D (i)
   E (ii)
   F (iv)

2 C It is unlikely that sufficient time would have lapsed to develop carbon monoxide (CO) poisoning; another cause must be considered.

3 E Note that pregnancy (answer D) *is* an indication for treatment because of the increased susceptibility of the fetus to CO.

Level 3: Topics for further discussion

1 Few centres have hyperbaric chambers on site, so careful allocation of resources is required before transport services are utilised to transfer patients. The Cochrane Library is a good place to start searching for current reviews on the use of hyperbaric oxygen therapy. In individual cases it is recommended that clinicians consult with a hyperbaric specialist to discuss treatment options.

2 This is the main reason that hyperbaric oxygen is recommended, but it can be difficult to quantify specific defects without specialised testing.

Case 6 review

Level 1: Content knowledge

1 A

2 B   A reduction in lung compliance due to dilution of surfactant is a major cause of the increase in the work of breathing seen in pulmonary oedema.

3 B   When inflammatory mediators circulate to the lungs they can alter the permeability of the pulmonary capillary endothelium.

Level 2: Clinical applications

1 D   BiPAP may increase myocardial workload and increase the rate of myocardial infarction in this circumstance; frusemide is still recommended even though its benefit does not occur for some hours post-administration

2 C   Hydralazine: this agent reduces afterload and can lead to rapid improvement in the patient's condition. D and E are contraindicated in acute decompensated heart failure

3 E   This would not be expected.

Level 3: Topics for further discussion

1 These two agents have been in use for many years, but are being superseded by the more widespread use of more effective therapies such as GTN and CPAP. Direct manipulation of the pathophysiological parameters seem to improve patient outcomes, and Level 1 evidence for their use is steadily appearing. Many emergency physicians see little role for morphine or frusemide in the acute management of pulmonary oedema for these reasons.

2 There are always two issues involved in the management of these patients: (a) treat the pulmonary oedema and (b) identify the precipitant. There are many potential precipitants, and timely use of bedside investigations (for example, the 12-lead ECG) may identify a range of treatable conditions.

Case 7 review

Level 1: Content knowledge

1 B   Volume overload upstream of the damaged ventricle is a key factor that enables hypovolaemic and cardiogenic shock to be differentiated.

2   C   Acidosis when severe can depress heart activity, further contributing to the shocked state.

3   D   An increase in preload will increase blood pressure to some degree in all forms of shock except for D.

Level 2: Clinical applications

1   C   Defibrillation is the only therapy of these proven to improve outcomes.

2   B   The combination of a witnessed cardiac arrest, early CPR and VF as the initial rhythm is associated with a relatively high rate of survival. The 'chain of survival' is maintained. The other scenarios have almost uniformly poor survival.

3   D   is not an indication for reperfusion, as defined in the ISIS 2 Study. Issues surrounding thrombolysis are covered in the recommended readings.

Level 3: Topics for further discussion

1   The 'chain of survival' is: Early access (that is, call an ambulance); Early CPR; Early defibrillation; and Early advanced cardiac life support (ACLS). A break in the chain can reduce survival. Many communities have addressed aspects of the chain by implementing community first aid programs and public access defibrillation.

2   There is a paucity of Level 1 evidence surrounding the management of patients in cardiac arrest. ACLS is a relatively new practice, having only been introduced in the form as we know it today in the 1960s. Up-to-date information is available from the International Liaison Committee on Resuscitation at www.c2005.org.

Case 8 review

Level 1: Content knowledge

1   B

2   D   Extrinsic asthma can be triggered by a range of common stimuli and lead to hypersensitivity, bronchial obstruction and mucosal oedema of the bronchioles.

3   A   Corticosteroids act by reducing bronchial hyperreactivity and inhibiting the release of mediators from cells induced by the inflammatory process.

Level 2: Clinical applications

1 C These patients are at risk of hypoxia and should receive a high concentration of inspired oxygen. Although an asthmatic may have impaired ventilation and hence an acute respiratory acidosis due to a high $PaCO_2$, this situation should not be confused with a patient with COPD in a similar situation: the asthmatic will not have a chronic respiratory acidosis that could suppress the ventilatory drive in the presence of excess oxygen.

2 **A** (iii)
  B (i)
  C (iv)
  D (ii)

3 C This is a reasonable PEF and implies only a mild exacerbation of asthma.

Level 3: Topics for further discussion

1 Asthma management plans allow exacerbations to be managed and for the anticipation of deterioration. Emergency Department staff need to liaise with local practitioners so that a coordinated management plan can be developed and implemented.

2 The use of non-invasive ventilation may have a role; other pharmacological interventions such as adrenaline, ketamine and volatile anaesthetic agents can be utilised in severe cases.

Case 9 review

Level 1: Content knowledge

1 B

2 B Chronic hypercapnia can reduce the sensitivity of the medullary chemoreceptors, leading to an overreliance on the hypoxic stimulation of peripheral chemoreceptors to regulate respiration. Oxygen therapy can therefore inadvertently remove or reduce the hypoxic stimulus to breathe.

3 B The $PaCO_2$ of arterial blood is inversely related to the degree of alveolar ventilation.

Level 2: Clinical applications

1 B The inspired oxygen concentration should be carefully titrated to achieve patient oxygen saturations between 88 and 92%. Caution

should be exercised when administering nebulisers—they should be attached to an air outlet rather than an oxygen outlet, in order to prevent excessive oxygen being administered.

2 **A** (ii)
   B (iii)
   C (iv)
   D (v)
   E (i)

3 D This represents an acute chronic respiratory acidosis, as would be expected in such a patient. B is an acute respiratory acidosis (as evidenced by the near-normal bicarbonate) and E represents a compensated chronic respiratory acidosis.

Level 3: Topics for further discussion

1 Non-invasive therapy has revolutionised the care of these patients in recent years, and all emergency clinicians should be familiar with its use. There may be a role for helium and oxygen ('Heliox') in management, but its use is still being defined. As outlined in the COPDX plan (Reference to Case 9: MJA 2003), prevention of exacerbations is of paramount importance.

2 30% of patients do not have a clear identifiable cause for their exacerbations, but antibiotics remain the mainstay of therapy. Antimicrobials should cover *Haemophilus influenzae*, *Streptococcus pneumoniae* and *Moraxella catarrhalis*. It is essential that local epidemiology and sensitivities be checked.

Case 10 review

Level 1: Content knowledge

1 E

2 A The neurological basis of major depression is poorly understood, but the best current explanation links depression with a deficit of monoamine neurotransmitters, noradrenaline and serotonin (also known as 5-Ht) in the forebrain.

3 D Inhibition of the reuptake of either noradrenaline or serotonin, or both, appears to be associated with antidepressant activity.

Level 2: Clinical applications

1 **A** (ii)
   B (iii)

C (v)
D (iv)
E (i)

2 B   An ECG is helpful in performing a risk assessment. A urinary drug screen rarely affects management.

3 D   Both staff and patient safety must be considered before resuscitation can commence.

4 **A** (iii)
   B (ii)
   C (v)
   D (i)
   E (iv)

5 E

6 B   This would be a feature of excessive muscarinic stimulation, not muscarinic blockade.

Level 3: Topics for further discussion

1 Clinical toxicologists are employed in a number of centres around the country and can offer a specialised advisory service. It is important that emergency departments have access to such information, as well as subscribing to various databases which can be used to guide therapy.

2 In the 21st century, terrorism is a threat in many countries of the world, and in the event of an incident, Emergency Departments provide the frontline medical response. Emergency Department staff need to be familiar with local disaster plans and appropriate medical responses to such potential incidents.

Case 11 review

Level 1: Content knowledge

1 C   An osmotic diuresis in DKA is caused by an elevated glucose loading in the nephrons of the kidney.

2 C   The acetone breath is caused by the elevated levels of ketone bodies in the pulmonary capillary blood tainting the alveolar gas.

3 D   Increasing the rate and depth of breathing will blow off more carbon dioxide and this will partially compensate for the metabolic acidosis associated with DKA.

Level 2: Clinical applications

1 C

2 B   Non-compliance is the most common precipitant

3 A   Cautious fluid resuscitation is recommended to prevent electrolyte disturbances and the possible development of cerebral oedema.

Level 3: Topics for further discussion

1 This is an important clinical issue, especially in children. Rapid correction of the blood glucose level is not recommended, so it is helpful to refer to various infusion guidelines for the management of these patients.

2 Diabetes is a condition where a team approach can improve outcomes. Collaboration between medical, nursing and allied health staff can provide a coordinated and comprehensive approach to young people with diabetes.

Case 12 review

Level 1: Content knowledge

1 C   Muscle damage can occur in rhabdomyolysis due to arterial occlusion (inadequate perfusion), direct compression leading to increased compartment pressure (disruption of cell membrane) or direct mechanical disruption of the cell.

2 A   In rhabdomyolysis, acute renal failure can often develop as a result of increased plasma haemoglobin and myoglobin levels and therefore the renal filtered load of these proteins.

3 D   Insulin, catecholamines, aldosterone and alkalosis all stimulate potassium uptake cells, therefore altering the internal balance of potassium.

Level 2: Clinical applications

1 B   Calcium gluconate acts as a cardiac stabiliser and may prevent dangerous arrhythmias forming as a result of hyperkalaemia.

2 A   As per the Cochrane review (Mahoney et al. 2005), this is the most effective intervention.

3 D   All of the other results are consistent with rhabdomyolysis.

Level 3: Topics for further discussion

1 Common electrolyte disturbances include disorders of sodium, potassium, and calcium. Their clinical presentations vary, but all can have serious consequences.

2 The emergency physician and the intensive care specialist need to prioritise and coordinate care; this requires practice and open communication between medical teams.

Integrated questions

1 A (iii) Tension pneumothorax, producing obstructive shock.
  B (i) Likely splenic injury producing haemorrhage leading to hypovolaemic shock.
  C (iii) Ventricular laceration producing pericardial tamponade: obstructive shock.
  D (ii) ECG diagnostic of acute myocardial infarction, therefore cardiogenic shock.
  E (iv) Anaphylaxis; distributive shock.
  F (i) Hypovolaemic shock, from excessive plasma loss (though internal injury should also be suspected if significant trauma occurs).
  G (i) Hypovolaemic shock from gastrointestinal blood loss, presumably from a bleeding peptic ulcer.
  H (iv) Distributive shock: loss of sympathetic tone leads to hypotension.
  I (iii) Pulmonary embolus must be considered: obstructive shock.
  J (i) Likely viral gastroenteritis leading to significant dehydration: hypovolaemic shock.
  K (iv) This clinical scenario is most likely meningococcal infection causing septic shock, and is a form of distributive shock. However, like anaphylaxis, other factors, such as suppression of myocardial contractility (producing cardiogenic shock), contribute to the shocked state.
2 B Blood gas analysis would not affect management in a child with asthma relieved simply by salbutamol. Painful procedures should be performed only if they are going to alter management.
3 A (iv)
  B (v)
  C (i)
  D (viii)
  E (vii)
4 A (ii)
  B (vi)
  C (iv)

D (iii)
E (vii)
F (i)
5 A (ii)
B (iii)
C (v)
D (i)
E (iv)
6 A (iv)
B (i)
C (ii)
D (v)
E (iii)
F (vi)

Index